Bob Guter
John R. Killacky
Editors

Queer Crips
Disabled Gay Men and Their Stories

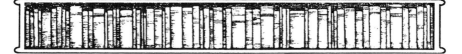

Queer Crips
Disabled Gay Men and Their Stories

HAWORTH Gay & Lesbian Studies
John P. De Cecco, PhD
Editor in Chief

Out of the Twilight: Fathers of Gay Men Speak by Andrew R. Gottlieb

The Mentor: A Memoir of Friendship and Gay Identity by Jay Quinn

Male to Male: Sexual Feeling Across the Boundaries of Identity by Edward J. Tejirian

Straight Talk About Gays in the Workplace, Second Edition by Liz Winfeld and Susan Spielman

The Bear Book II: Further Readings in the History and Evolution of a Gay Male Subculture edited by Les Wright

Gay Men at Midlife: Age Before Beauty by Alan L. Ellis

Being Gay and Lesbian in a Catholic High School: Beyond the Uniform by Michael Maher

Finding a Lover for Life: A Gay Man's Guide to Finding a Lasting Relationship by David Price

The Man Who Was a Woman and Other Queer Tales from Hindu Lore by Devdutt Pattanaik

How Homophobia Hurts Children: Nurturing Diversity at Home, at School, and in the Community by Jean M. Baker

The Harvey Milk Institute Guide to Lesbian, Gay, Bisexual, Transgender, and Queer Internet Research edited by Alan Ellis, Liz Highleyman, Kevin Schaub, and Melissa White

Stories of Gay and Lesbian Immigration: Together Forever? by John Hart

From Drags to Riches: The Untold Story of Charles Pierce by John Wallraff

Lyton Strachey and the Search for Modern Sexual Identity: The Last Eminent Victorian by Julie Anne Taddeo

Before Stonewall: Activists for Gay and Lesbian Rights in Historical Context edited by Vern L. Bullough

Sons Talk About Their Gay Fathers: Life Curves by Andrew R. Gottlieb

Restoried Selves: Autobiographies of Queer Asian/Pacific American Activists edited by Kevin K. Kumashiro

Queer Crips: Disabled Gay Men and Their Stories by Bob Guter and John R. Killacky

Dirty Young Me and Other Gay Stories by Joseph Itiel

Queering Creole Spiritual Traditions: Lesbian, Gay, Bisexual, and Transgender Participation in African-Inspired Traditions in the Americas by Randy P. Conner with David Hatfield Sparks

How It Feels to Have a Gay or Lesbian Parent: A Book by Kids for Kids of All Ages by Judith E. Snow

Queer Crips
Disabled Gay Men and Their Stories

Bob Guter
John R. Killacky
Editors

HPP

Harrington Park Press®
An Imprint of The Haworth Press, Inc.
New York • London • Oxford

Published by

Harrington Park Press®, an imprint of The Haworth Press, Inc., 10 Alice Street, Binghamton, NY 13904-1580.

Cover design by Jennifer M. Gaska.

Library of Congress Cataloging-in-Publication Data

Queer crips : disabled gay men and their stories / Bob Guter, John R. Killacky, editors.
    p. cm.
    ISBN 1-56023-456-3 (hard cover : alk. paper)—ISBN 1-56023-457-1 (soft cover : alk. paper)
    1. Gay men—Interviews. 2. People with disabilities—Interviews. I. Guter, Bob. II. Killacky, John R.
    HQ76.Q423 2003
    305.38'9664—dc21
                                                    2002154812

For
G. O. and Larry Connolly

CONTENTS

ABOUT THE EDITORS

Bob Guter created *BENT: A Journal of Cripgay Voices* in 1999, and continues to edit and manage the influential webzine. *BENT* has been excerpted by the *Utne Reader* and praised by the Annenberg School of Communication's *Online Journalism Review.* Guter last spoke on queer/disability issues at the first International Queer Disability Conference in San Francisco. He has written for *The New York Times, Stagebill,* and *New Jersey History.*

John R. Killacky is a former dancer, ex-marathon runner, now paraplegic. By day he is an arts administrator, at night he writes personal narrative, and on weekends he makes videos aspiring to be visual poems. His work has been anthologized in *Queer Dharma* and *Out in All Directions,* and has appeared in numerous publications, including the *Utne Reader,* the *San Francisco Examiner, Art Papers,* the *Hungry Mind Review,* the *Bay Area Reporter, Inside Arts,* and *Disability Studies Quarterly.*

Contributors

Raymond J. Aguilera holds a BA in English from the University of California, Berkeley, and is a graduate student in human sexuality studies at San Francisco State, where he is researching relationships between disabled and nondisabled partners. Ray once spilled chamomile tea on Allen Ginsberg.

J. Quinn Brisben, a retired Chicago high school teacher, has been active in progressive causes since the 1950s. His recent Atlanta arrest was his eighth with ADAPT, his fifteenth in a social cause. In 1990 he and his wife took 3,000 condoms from ACT/UP Chicago to the Moscow Gay and Lesbian Union.

Eli Clare is a transgendered poet, rabble rouser, and author of *Exile and Pride: Disability, Queerness, and Liberation,* South End Press, 1999.

Walt Dudley was born in North Dakota in 1952. He lived in the Netherlands, was schooled briefly in Nairobi, then followed music scholarships around the United States. Since his MS diagnosis in 1975, he has written and spoken frequently on disability issues. His book *We're the People, Too,* can be found at <www.championpress. com>.

Gordon Elkins was born in Oklahoma in 1945 and contracted polio at age eight, six months before the Salk vaccine was available. He has worked for social change as a community activist involved in many service organizations. His two adopted gay sons are his pride and joy.

Robert Feinstein's writing has appeared in the gay French Canadian magazine *RG* and the *Utne Reader* online. In his many articles for *BENT* he hopes to "convey the realities of life as a blind gay man." Bob lives with his guide dog Harley in Brooklyn, New York.

Kenny Fries, author of *Body, Remember: A Memoir* (Dutton, 1997), and editor of *Staring Back: The Disability Experience from the Inside Out* (Plume, 1997), is a recipient of the Gregory Kolovakos Award and the Japan/US Creative Arts Program Grant. *Desert Walking* (Advocado Press, 2000) is his new book of poems. He teaches at Goddard College.

Ed Gallagher was born in 1957. A former college jock, he became a writer, lecturer, and the host of his own TV talk show after suffering a spinal cord injury in 1985. His three books are published under the aegis of his foundation, Alive to Thrive, Inc., in New Rochelle, New York <www.alivetothrive.org>.

J. Douglas George is a raconteur, bon vivant, and generally fun guy to have around. He's been a poet and a thief, though usually not at the same time. For now, he's content to look out the window and watch the trees grow.

Carmelo Gonzalez lives in Manhattan, where he writes prose and poetry influenced by his experience with cerebral palsy. Find out more about his life and work at <www.carmelo418.com>.

Chris Hewitt's poems and translations have appeared in *The New Yorker, The American Poetry Review, The Advocate,* and *The James White Review.* He has "brittle bone disease" (osteogenesis imperfecta) and has gotten around in a wheelchair since he was nine.

Born and raised in Los Angeles, **Danny Kodmur** studied history at Stanford and UC Berkeley. He writes and speaks frequently about disability and sexuality, and is thrilled that this anthology, his book debut, is parked at their intersection. In a blue space, of course.

A disability pension from the New York City Transit Authority enabled **Donald H. Lawrence Jr.** to escape from the Big Apple to the tranquility of a small town in North Carolina, where he shares his life and home with his Aunt Lois, two dogs, three cats, and, recently and miraculously, his once cyber-, now actual lover, Bruce.

Raymond Luczak's five books include *Eyes of Desire: A Deaf Gay & Lesbian Reader* (Alyson), *St. Michael's Fall: Poems* (Deaf Life Press), *Silence Is a Four-Letter Word: On Art and Deafness, This Way to the Acorns: Poems,* and *Snooty: A Comedy* (the last three from Tactile Mind Press). He wrote and directed his debut feature film *Ghosted.* His Web site is <www.raymondluczak.com>.

Samuel Lurie is a queer transman who lives in Vermont and travels nationally providing transgender awareness training to health care providers. His relationship with a knockout crip/tranny/queer boy has taught him an unquantifiable amount about overcoming shame, learning new ways to love, and about staying calm while leaping off high cliffs.

Thomas Metz lives with his partner, David Brightman, in San Francisco. Tom has performed with Axis Dance Company and the Lake Merrymen Players. He has written for newspapers, magazines, and *A Family and Friends' Guide to Sexual Orientation* (Routledge Press, 1996), as well as for corporate clients in Silicon Valley.

Karl Michalak (1958-1997), MFA Columbia University, was a writer, artist, singer-songwriter, film critic, performance artist, and political activist. During his life he had a dozen operations to correct congenital physical anomalies. Information about a memorial CD of Karl's songs is available at <eoel@mindspring.com>.

Lorenzo W. Milam is retired and living in Guatemala and other south-of-the-border countries. His books include *The Cripple Liberation Front Marching Band Blues, Sex and Broadcasting,* and *Cripzen: A Manual for Survival.* Lorenzo got polio at age sixteen.

Mark Moody began writing in January 1998 in response to his first cancer diagnosis. He has survived two more bouts with cancer, as well as seventeen years with HIV. His poems have appeared in *a&u, The James White Review,* and online in *BENT.* He lives in Baltimore.

Michael Perreault had polio in infancy and embraced his gayness in his twenties. "I seldom felt part of the disabled community because I was gay," he writes, "or the gay community because I was disabled. Middle age has been about reconciling those contradictions within myself."

George Steven Powell lives in the wilds of East Texas, though his imagination ranges far afield—as his Web page <www.geocities. com/royalstu/index.html> attests. His stories have appeared in *Advocate Men, Freshmen, Honcho, Inches, Play Guy, Options,* and other magazines.

Since his birth in 1968, **Joel S. Riche** has been disabled by an undiagnosed nerve disorder that affects his balance and coordination. He went to both undergraduate and law school at UC Berkeley. He has practiced law in San Francisco and Los Angeles. He lives in West Hollywood.

Robert I. Roth is chief executive officer of the Deaf Counseling, Advocacy and Referral Agency of San Leandro, California, and often provides presentations on deaf artists, art criticism, and arts access. He has been published in several anthologies of stories about the deaf community.

Alan Sable, a San Francisco psychotherapist primarily serving the gay community, was perhaps the first out gay professor in the United States. Due to this he lost his academic position in 1977. He holds a BA from Stanford and an MA and PhD from Harvard. At sixty-one years old he is thus far physically fully abled.

Alex Sendham lives in Colorado in comforting proximity to virtually everyone named in his work. Some names, he concedes, have been changed to protect the rueful. He has been paraplegic since 1968.

Steven Sickles was born in California in 1954 and finally had the sense to move back in 1989. He has a BA in fine art with a minor in art history. In 1996 he developed meningitis, which left his right hand fingerless. He lives in Los Angeles with his new husband, Dan.

Born in the Bronx fifty-three years ago, **Max E. Verga** lived a life of quiet desperation until he learned that the pen is mightier than the sword. As causes tumbled into his lap, he learned that the worst thing you can say about anyone is the truth, and the best that you can say is that everyone deserves to hear that truth.

Greg Walloch coproduced and stars in *Fuck the Disabled,* and is featured in three other films: John Killacky's *Crip Shots,* Burn Manhattan's *Clean,* and Larry Ferber's *Cruise Control.* Greg's live show, "White Disabled Talent," tours the United States, the United Kingdom, Australia, and Ireland. He has appeared off Broadway at Joe's Pub at The Public Theater.

Blaine Waterman is a librarian with cerebral palsy and a writer whose work has appeared in *The Encyclopedia of Gay and Lesbian Literature, Able-Together,* and online in *BENT.*

Preface

This is a book full of characters, drama, conflict, narrative—in short, a book of stories. Storytelling begins as an intimate act. It's a solo turn, a reflection of our own innermost feelings, but inside the stories we tell dwells another impulse, the desire to connect.

We not only tell stories, we listen, too, to the stories of others. If we are fortunate, our elders enrich us with versions of the family saga that are frequently funny, sometimes tragic, and often mysteriously contradictory, stories that help us recognize the evanescent nature of personal truth.

We are enthralled by the stories of our friends and bound inextricably to our lovers by stories that begin as pillow talk and end up becoming the stories that weave our lives together.

All of us are capable of telling stories in different ways and to different audiences, but the same handful of reasons for telling them remains constant. We tell stories to create our selves, and sometimes to transform our understanding of ourselves. We create personal narrative to defend those selves from attack, to confirm our membership in the tribe (however defined), and to invite the approval and love of others.

The best stories are resilient in the face of repetition. We want to hear them over and over because they comfort us. They help us to know one another in a deeper way. The most compelling stories, both those we tell and those we hear, are the ones that get embedded for life somewhere deep inside us.

But what does storytelling in general have to do with being queer and disabled?

The point is painfully simple: Although all of us have stories and all of us are capable of telling stories, we can also be disenfranchised from the stories of our own lives, censored by bias and public opinion, silenced by oppressive institutions from within (the family), or from without (church and state). When this happens we risk becoming nonpersons. We end up in a kind of Gulag of the self, where we ourselves don't know who we are.

In the past twenty years or so we have all seen the avalanche of queer-themed books—popular, academic, and pulp—that has helped to give us a public identity and a common culture; but disabled people, especially queer disabled people, have not participated in the same phenomenon. Because we are a minority within a minority, a niche market, in advertising speak, we will never find our stories overflowing the shelves at Barnes & Noble, or even at A Different Light. Maybe that's not such a loss, since commodification can do a lot of damage to minority culture.

There's a bigger problem, however, one we need to face up to. As queer crips, we've been isolated from society at large and even from one another, by underemployment, institutionalization, poverty, and internalized cripophobia. All these factors have not merely discouraged us from telling our stories, they have brainwashed us into believing we have no stories to tell. The result is far more insidious than being unable to find ourselves remaindered at the local bookstore. What happens is that we, ourselves, fail to construct our own narratives. Fearing we are wordless, it becomes easy for us to believe we are worthless.

Discouraged from fashioning our own stories, we find we have no stories to share, even with our peers. We cease to exist not only as individuals true to ourselves but as people with things in common, and thus we lack a common culture.

If the Big World, the mainstream, refuses to recognize us, there's only one thing to do: create our own narrative ways and means. That is the purpose of this anthology. It is both a refuge and a billboard for neglected cripgay voices. It proves that we do have something to say and that we know how to say it. The rewards for all of us who find ourselves in these pages are enormous. Talking to one another, and to you who read our words, grants us power and a place in the world.

Our words are candid, edgy, bold, dreamy, challenging, and sexy. What more could you ask from a good story?

Bob Guter

My journey with this book began seven years ago. Spinal surgery gone awry short-circuited my body permanently. In my initial frenzy and shock, I had no frame of reference. Remarking to my doctor how sorry I felt for Christopher Reeve because he was paralyzed, she looked surprised and asked, "What do you think you are?"

In rehab, I worked alongside patients dealing with strokes or brain and spinal injuries. I resisted being in a group situation—not wanting to identify with others, feeling safer in my own isolation. Seeing people worse off made me feel less sorry for myself— that is, until someone more flexible and mobile showed up.

In-house psychologists and social workers tried their best to be empathetic and supportive, although none could explain sexual functioning after spinal injury through a queer lens. Not one of them understood that this should be part of their job description, regardless of their own sexual orientation.

Out of the hospital, I was greeted with alarmed expressions and open-mouthed pity and treated as totally helpless. More than once my husband was asked how I was feeling as he pushed me along in a wheelchair. I ignored sympathetic smiles from the more fully abled and sought out eye contact with members of my new tribe. I longed to meet other gay men who were disabled.

I found comfort reading Lorenzo W. Milam's *Cripple Liberation Front Marching Band Blues* (Mho & Mho Works), Kenny Fries' *Staring Back* (Plume), Reynolds Price's *A Whole New Life* (Scribner Classics), and Raymond Luczak's *Eyes of Desire* (Alyson). While I did not know other queer crips, at least I was not alone. Eventually I began to meet and network with other like-bodied men.

I first came across coeditor Bob Guter's work in *Able-Together,* a quarterly 'zine for men with disabilities. I became more of a fan through his *Bent: A Journal of Cripgay Voices,* a powerful and empowering Web 'zine for disabled queer men. Together we joined forces to compile this collection of writings. The list of contributors grew organically through our contacts and as one writer suggested another. E-mail buddies further spread the word as our literary community developed.

In this anthology, you will read first-person accounts by men with cerebral palsy, muscular dystrophy, post-polio syndrome, spinal cord injury, deafness, blindness, spina bifida, osteogenesis imperfecta, AIDS, amputation, congenital damage, and traumatic injury and disfigurement, as well as unnamed mobility and neuromuscular disorders.

Together we present *Queer Crips: Disabled Gay Men and Their Stories.*

John R. Killacky

Acknowledgments

No thanks on my part can repay the emotional generosity of the men whose stories make up this book. George Taleporos invited me to write "Destination *Bent*" for a special issue of *Sexuality and Disability*. His insights were critical in shaping the piece; Jean Stewart and Tom Metz helped refine its ideas and language. Mark McBeth's creative and technical support made a rough road smooth.

B. G.

For their grace, generosity, and connectivity in shaping the anthology, I am grateful to Tim Miller, Barry Corbet, Kippy Stroud, and all the queer crips.

J. R. K.

The following chapters, sometimes in slightly different form, appeared in *Bent: A Journal of Cripgay Voices* (www.bentvoices.org). Authors hold individual copyright in all cases.

- Raymond J. Aguilera, "The Boy I Used to Be" (January 2002)
- J. Quinn Brisben, "A Wedding Celebration" (November 2001)
- Walt Dudley, "Homo on the Range" (January 2001)
- Robert Feinstein, "Alone in the Crowd" (July 2000)
- J. Douglas George, "Becoming Daddy's Boy" (March 2001)
- Carmelo Gonzalez, an excerpt from Chapter Three of *Rolling On* (May 2002). This is a radically edited and condensed version of Chapter 3 of the author's self-published memoir, *Rolling On.* Copyright 2001.
- Bob Guter and Alan Sable, "How to Find Love with a Fetishist" (May 2001)
- Bob Guter, Thomas Metz, and Michael Perreault, "Dancing Toward the Light" (July 2000)
- Chris Hewitt, "Sticks and Stones" (November 2000); Four poems: "The Lifting Team" (January 2001), "Reincarnation," and "Skimming" (September 2001); "What Brains Are For" (December 1999)
- Danny Kodmur, "On Being (Un)Representative" (January 2002)
- Don Lawrence, "Queer Ducks" (January 2002)
- Thomas Metz, "Love Is All Around" (July 2001)
- Mark Moody, "Persistence, Memory" (May 2000)
- Michael Perreault, "Acting for Others, Acting for Myself" (January 2001)
- George Steven Powell, "But I Don't Like You Like That" (December 1999)
- Steven Sickles, "Working It Out" (December 2001)
- Max E. Verga, "A Meeting with George Dureau" (July 2000)

Two Performance Pieces

Greg Walloch

WALKING

Lights up. Performer enters walking on crutches and dressed in white briefs. Performer walks back and forth across the stage, then stops and speaks.

When I was about twelve or thirteen, my parents took me to the local medical clinic. When I got to the clinic I was asked to strip down to my underwear and after awhile a nurse would call me into the main room.

In the main room sat a panel of about thirty-five people: doctors, therapists, and students. The nurse would give me my cue to begin, and I would walk back and forth in front of the panel. Sometimes one of the doctors would stop me, then move his hand down my back, grab my ankle, or poke at one of my ribs. I would wait until he was done, and begin to walk again as the panel took notes. They would just stare at me, make an occasional medical comment, and take more notes.

I walked in front of this panel for an hour. Actually walking out in front of the panel was the easy part. The difficult part was all the time beforehand, all that time waiting. I was really afraid of what those thirty-five people might think.

When I got to the clinic, a nurse would lead me to a small room in the back of the building. This room had white walls and a white tile floor. Above the door was a big wall clock, and in the corner was a folding metal chair. I would sit on the metal chair in my underwear, staring at the clock, and I would pray. Only five minutes to go. Please don't let it happen. . . . Please don't let it happen! And then I would look down, and sure enough, I would have the biggest erection I've ever had in my entire life! I'd put it to the left, I'd put it to the right. Up! Then down! Left . . . then right . . . God, nothing looks right!

Then a nurse would come in, and she would say: "Mr. Walloch, you can come in now."

Performer stands and walks back and forth across the stage. Stops downstage in front of chair. Soften lights slightly.

My brother and I went into Denny's one night about 2:45 a.m. It was pretty empty, there were a couple of people sitting around; most of them were men. We sat down and the waitress came over to our table to take our order. She looked to my brother to take his order, but he wasn't very hungry, he didn't want anything. Then the waitress looked to me; "I'd like a glass of milk and a slice of strawberry pie." The waitress took this down and went to the kitchen.

Just then this big guy walked in with his girlfriend. He said: "Would you look at all the fuckin' faggots in Denny's tonight! Goddamn it, you can't fuckin' go anywhere without seeing a faggot these days!" This man and his girlfriend were seated at the table across from mine. When they sat down, he looked up at me and said: "I'm looking at you, you fag! I'm looking at you, you fuckin' queer! Come on, come on. I saw you looking at me when I walked in. I saw you look at me. Come on, you fucking queer! Come on, I saw you looking at me; you queers are always looking at me! You can sit there and pretend you don't hear me, but I know you hear me, faggot! You'd better watch your ass in that parking lot man! I'm gonna fuckin' kill you, man!"

By this time my brother had made a quick escape to the bathroom. I tried to sit calmly and finish eating. "Come on you fuckin' queer, look at me. I know you want to look at me. Lift up your fuckin' head and look!" Then the guy turns to his girlfriend and says: "You see that faggot over there? Do you see that fag? I am going to kill him for you! I'm gonna kill that faggot just for you!"

And I thought: You know? What better way could there be to impress your date?

"I hate you fuckin' queers and I'm going to kill every one of you! You'd better watch your fuckin' ass, man, because next time you look around, I'm going to be the one behind you!" The other people at Denny's were trying quite hard to ignore what was going on. I decided to go see the manager. I get up and the man and his girlfriend move from their table. The man walks toward me and he puts his hand on my shoulder and says: "Aw, man, fuck . . . I'm sorry. I mean . . .

I didn't . . . I didn't know that you were fucked up like that. I didn't know that you were crippled and shit. You can't be a fag."

Performer walks back and forth across the stage. Stops upstage behind chair, leans on chair back. Soften lights slightly.

Not long ago I was part of a panel at a university. The university called it The Day of Understanding. The idea here was to discuss sexuality on both a personal and social level. I felt very vulnerable that day, like anybody could ask me anything. There were some interesting questions. "When did you first know that you were gay? What was it like to realize that?" or "How has AIDS and the fear of AIDS affected your lives and what you do?" Then one guy asked: "How does it feel to kiss another guy? I mean to have his tongue in your mouth, and does it feel really weird if you both haven't shaved?"

Then a woman stood up in the back and addressed me: "I have a comment for the man on the end. I've been listening to you today, and I think that you are a bright and intelligent young man gone very wrong. You have to understand that the choice that you have made in your life is a sin. Your body is crippled, because it is crippled with sin. Don't you see? If you go to church God will help you. God can heal you. God gave you a disability, because he knew that you were going to be gay. Now don't take offense at what I'm saying. If you make the right choice, God can heal you. If you just make the choice to change your lifestyle, God can help you in so many ways. Only then will you become a true servant to God and be his divine gift. Know that what you do in your life is a sin, and I don't have a question for you. I just want to know, are you going to accept God as your savior?"

Performer walks back and forth across the stage. Stops downstage right, close to audience. Soften lights slightly. Sharpen focus on chair.

I saw you walking around out here, and I just wanted to ask you: "What happened to you?" I also wanted to tell you that I think that you are such an inspiration. . . . You are so beautiful and full of light. I knew this guy once that had the same problem. Maybe you know him? To see you put so much effort into something like walking, something I take for granted. You are so brave and full of courage; it must be really hard. You're special, and don't you ever forget that somebody up there loves you. You don't ever have to worry. I'll think of you; you will be in my prayers. You are truly an inspiration to every one of us.

FUCK THE DISABLED

I was sitting at brunch with a friend of mine. She said, "Greg, can I ask you a personal question?" and I said, "Sure," because you know, I'm very open that way. She said, "Is the reason that you're gay due to the fact that you're crippled and you can't get lucky with women, so you had no other choice but to sleep with men for sex? You know, I was just wondering."

I looked at her and was like: "Are you reading my mind? I was just thinking about that! Yes, that is *exactly* the reason I sleep with men. It's a sad story, my life. You see, underneath it all I'm actually a heterosexual man, but because of my unfortunate, grotesque disfigurement I was shunned by women and polite society and forced into the depravity of the underground world of man-to-man sex. I never much cared for sucking dick, but if I wanted any action I had better get used to it . . . and all the while, in my chest beat the heart of a broken man."

My friend's like: "That's nice, Greg. Can you pass the butter?"

I explained to her that it was a matter of economics and weighing my options at the time. Should I waste my money on expensive female prostitutes or be gay? Instead of spending my money on expensive hookers, I found I could get free sex from gay men who had a discriminating eye for fashion, but not for sexual partners. I decided that being gay was cheaper, but I had no idea about the hidden costs: the parades, the clothes, the expensive party drugs . . . not to mention the apartment in Chelsea, a pretty daunting political agenda, and the painful anal shenanigans. Ouch!

I never wanted to be gay. I tried to fight it, but soon I found I'd developed a strange addiction to crack . . . a different kind of crack. You know, the sacrifices that the disabled have to make in this country today because of lack of acceptance are unbelievable! If you're disabled, don't make the same mistakes I did. Don't let this happen to you.

That's why I started my own foundation called "Fuck the Disabled." So if you're a woman eighteen to thirty-five and you would like to "Fuck the Disabled," call us at 212-DIS-ABLE.

Are you attracted to subservient men? Well, crippled guys can barely stand up. Have you had bizarre sexual fantasies involving a midget or several midgets? We can help. And you know what they say about mentally retarded men? Small intellect, big . . . you know what I'm talking about.

So call us: 212-DIS-ABLE. Fuck the Disabled to keep the disabled from turning gay.

Hustlers: A Buyer's Guide

Blaine Waterman

Throughout my twenties I didn't have an awful lot of luck with sex. I was horny all the time. I thought about calling a hustler, but the idea made me nervous. Not out of a sense that it was wrong or bad— I just had a lot of anxiety about exactly what the interaction would be like, what kind of person would show up at my door if I called. So I didn't explore it until late in 1994, when I was thirty years old. I had a boyfriend then, but our sexual relationship was kind of not there; we were still warm and friendly, but sexually, for whatever reason, it was going nowhere. I just decided I wanted sex, specifically with younger, cute guys, the kind of guys I'd never had success attracting on my own.

So I started to call hustlers, mostly from ads in the *Bay Area Reporter,* because they publish photos there and people seemed pretty accessible and it was easy to find lots of choices. The first guy I called was nice enough, but not my type. It was awkward. He actually showed up when Greg, one of my helpers, was on his way out. I told Greg, "Oh, yeah, I called up this hustler; he's gonna come over," and Greg, who's straight, thought it was pretty funny. So this guy comes in and he was like "Tenderloiny"; his hair was a real fake blond. He was not horribly unattractive or anything, but I just wasn't that into him. And he obviously was not that into doing anything. I found later that some of the guys are pretty horny themselves and seem to like the sex as much as the money. But he was not in that club. He was obviously into delivering as little as possible for the money. So what I ended up doing was having him give me a bath. We didn't have sex at all! He gave me a bath and I talked to him about being a hustler.

My second experience was on a trip with a friend to LA. I was looking in *Frontiers* and saw an ad for a guy named Troy Steel. My friend said, "Yeah, he's got a really great body. Call him up." So I did. He was a nice guy and I was pretty attracted to him, a lot more than the first guy, but he was not into affection at all, not into kissing, only sucking and fucking. I think I gave Troy a blow job and he gave me a blow job, and we hung around his house and he showed me some of his glossies (he was some kind of minor porn star). He signed one of the glossies. I've shown it to a lot of people. So in some ways that was one of my more fun experiences, although he wasn't all that affectionate, like kissy-face, and I didn't come or anything. But it was fun because it was the Hollywood thing and he was sort of a character. I mean he was a nice guy. He wasn't a mean person or anything. I think he had drawn a line for himself that he wasn't going to cross and kissing, for him, was on the other side of the line.

Although I didn't fully realize it at the time, I don't have any fun unless there's some expression of affection, unless there's some kind of huggy-kissy action. If all they want to do is get it over with, for me it doesn't work, although I know that's what a lot of guys want. It took me a while (duh!) to figure that out for myself. That's one of the ways that buying hustlers was good for me in kind of an educational way. Aside from whatever fun (or not) I had with them, the experience got me a little more in touch with what I wanted, or needed, from people.

When you stop to think about it, if you're expecting affection, or at least a simulation of affection, I guess that that might be more difficult for most hustlers than the old in and out. I think it's easier for the hustler to depersonalize hustling when he's just letting a guy fuck him, say, when he's basically just being an orifice. Kissing is real personal. There were a lot of hustlers who made kissing an optional thing for them. After I learned that's what I wanted, I'd make a point of asking over the phone, "Do you kiss?" or, "Do you let guys kiss you?" And they might say, "It depends." I guess what it depended on was whether they thought you were fairly cute, or had a nice personality, I'm not sure exactly what, but at least you knew from the start that they weren't automatically going to rule it out. No one who said, "it depends" ever turned me down for kissing, which, of course, felt good. But it took me several encounters before I realized that I had to ask for what I wanted, or I was going to end up feeling bitter and frustrated.

One kid, whose hustling name was Zack, I ended up calling a bunch of times. He was really cute; at least I thought so: short blond hair, lots of tattoos and piercings. Maybe the best thing about him, though, was that he loved to kiss; that was his favorite thing to do.

Expectations are the thing. I mean, if a hustler was very cute and very friendly with me, I was disappointed if he didn't get off. After a while I began to add up my expectations and realized what was making me unhappy about hiring hustlers was that I wanted a boyfriend. And a hustler is never a boyfriend, simple as that. No matter how sweet, or cute, or nice he is, he's not your boyfriend. He's providing a service you're paying for, which is something you might want to forget. Part of the reason I wanted a hustler to come if I really was attracted to him was so that I could tell myself he was enjoying it as much as I was.

I don't regret seeing hustlers, but I think it took me a year or more to figure out what my real feelings were. The bottom line is, I hadn't been able to separate the desire for love from being horny, and I think some people can separate them. Maybe the line is always blurry, maybe some people can separate the two some of the time, but I wasn't able to separate them at all, even to the point of being semifriends with a couple of hustlers.

There were two in particular, Tim, and another guy, Richard, both of whom expressed an interest in doing things with me other than getting paid for sex. I went to a movie with Tim once. He helped me move from one apartment to another, so we were friendly, but then it ended, I think partly because of the tensions in the hustler-client relationship. With the client, there's the tension between wanting to be loved but knowing you're just paying for sex. With hustlers, some want to be loved or liked for themselves, apart from their sexual marketability. There's some touchiness there if they feel there's any confusion about that. With Tim, I really did like him as a person, but I was also horny and wanted sex with him. I think he wanted our relationship to change from my being one of his johns to being one of his friends. But I wanted to mix and match. As things developed, I guess I wanted to turn him into a boyfriend, someone I fucked because I liked him. Although he never said so, I'm convinced now that he found that disturbing, confusing.

With the second guy, Richard, a similar thing happened, although I never did as much with him. Richard also showed interest in spending time with me apart from being paid. Then I called him once when I was really horny and wanted to have sex, and he said, "Well, I really need money." So I said, "OK, just come over and I'll pay you because I like you a whole lot." So he came and saw me as a client. That

seemed alright at the time, but our friendship never really went anywhere after that.

One other thing I learned to do was mention being disabled when I
called a guy for the first time. Nobody seemed to have a problem with
it. One thing surprised me: I expected it to be a fairly common
experience—I mean for hustlers to deal with disabled clients—but I
found out it was not. I knew that a lot of hustlers see older guys (although I learned that the client range is a lot wider than I thought), but
very few had had a disabled client. A couple of times it was a problem, and then it was very awkward. I had this one real young Asian
guy, maybe nineteen or twenty, come over. He was one of the most attractive hustlers I ever met, and boy did he need therapy. He'd had a
cousin who died of muscular dystrophy. Even though I don't have
that, I reminded him of his cousin. He was also one of the few hustlers
I met who was up-front in his ambivalence about what he was doing.
We ended up not having sex. In fact, I guess I played therapist. That
was one of the few times I regretted the whole thing, even though I
felt sorry for him. Later I felt like a fool. I mean, I ended up paying
him $120; he should have paid me!

I'm still curious that none of my hustlers had any other disabled
clients. Maybe I've overestimated the need that disabled gay men
might have to hire hustlers. Maybe it's not as common an impulse as I
thought. But I know there's a lot of social isolation among disabled
gay men; a lot of us aren't out mixing. Maybe some guys don't do it
because, even though they're paying for it, it does take a certain bold-
ness. After all, I was afraid to pick up the phone for ten years.

Another factor is money. A lot of seriously disabled guys are on
SSI, and let's face it, buying a hustler is not like buying a six-pack;
low-income guys don't have the means to buy luxury items such as a
$100 whore. One of the many reasons I cut down and then gave up on
hustlers was the money. I'm employed, but the cost adds up. For a
while I was using guys twice a month.

But my other reasons are probably more important. Not only is
there the embarrassment, there's also the fear. How do you know
what kind of person you're inviting into your house? I guess I've been
lucky. Apart from some guys not performing very well (the limp dick
problem), I've never been ripped off and I've never run into someone
I was afraid of.

You've also got to remember that simply because you're paying for it doesn't mean that things are going to go the way you want them to. Just handing the guy money does not guarantee anything. You may think that in a sense you're buying a commodity, but it's not a dish detergent. There's only so much you can buy from another person, and then the human element overtakes everything else. In that way, buying the services of a hustler isn't any different from hiring the services of a masseur, a doctor, or a lawyer. If the client and the lawyer don't have at least some minimal degree of human compatibility, it's not going to be very satisfactory.

Another thing I learned about hustlers was that they weren't very together people—big surprise! Many used drugs, many were abandoned by their families. Drama always lurked in the background, lots of drama. The one boy, Tim, with whom I became sort of friends, claimed he had none of those things, and that seemed to be the case. He was bright, he was employed, he was good-looking, but he seemed pretty lonely. That's sad and disturbing. Here's somebody I'm hiring for sex, somebody who looks to me like he's "got everything," and it turns out he's no happier or better adjusted than I am.

The other danger is the danger of disease or infection of some kind, even if you're doing your best to play safe. The worst thing that happened to me was scabies, and yes, it's as bad as people say it is. No, it's worse! It's a nightmare.

On an even more serious level, I pretty much always had condoms ready to use. There was one guy, though, who was not very concerned about safe sex. He wanted me to fuck him without a condom, and I went along with it for a few minutes. But then we weren't connecting very well and I stopped. In retrospect I can't believe I did it. I'm not a dummy. I know all about safe sex. I got tested a couple of times afterward and never did anything like it again, but it was a disturbing episode. The point is that even if you're well-informed, it's easy to be stupid when you're horny, lonely, and with someone you want to like you. This boy was really cute and within seconds my resolve crumbled.

When I first started buying sex I was curious about prostitution, but when I think about it now, I think my hustler days are probably over, because, as I said earlier, I discovered that hustlers can't deliver what I'm after. Over a period of eighteen months (and about twenty guys), I learned a lot about it. And I learned a lot about myself in the process.

Sticks and Stones

Chris Hewitt

> Sticks and stones
> may break my bones,
> but names will
> never hurt me.

Children's Rhyme

If you're in a wheelchair, nondisabled people seem to feel they can come up to you on the street, in the park, on a bus—just about anywhere—and comment about your appearance. It's as if the chair turns the person in it into an invulnerable, insensitive object with no feelings, no reactive, normal human qualities.

Several times ushers in movie theaters have said to me, "You can't park in the aisle. You're a fire hazard!" Whenever I'm assaulted like this, I am shocked, amused, and angered all at once. I always think of a witty riposte minutes, hours, or even days later. I might have told the usher, "Well, I may be a flaming queen, but I'm not about to burn the house down!" Of course, anyone who makes a remark like that in the first place is not likely to get the joke. Here in San Francisco I've been the recipient of more rude and obnoxious comments from straight people than from gay people. Maybe gay people identify more easily with someone who represents another kind of minority.

On the other hand, I have been harassed most relentlessly by African-American school kids and teenagers. One kid, about fifteen, came up to me on Castro Street in the heart of gay San Francisco and said, "Do me a favor, willya?" "Sure," I replied. "Next Christmas tell Santa I want a new bicycle." I couldn't make sense of this at first. Later I realized he was addressing me as if I were one of Santa's elves.

I wish I could think of appropriate replies when I am accosted in this way. I'd like the kids to learn who and what I am, but on a noisy city street it would be difficult to explain it to them; it's unlikely that they would even hear me over all their laughter and commotion. White kids, as a rule, react timidly: They whisper among themselves and point at me. I might hear an occasional "midget" or "dwarf," but nothing more.

Adults can be equally rude. Once I was in line for a movie when a gold-chain-bedecked young man turned to his girlfriend and announced, "I don't wanna go ta this movie theater; it's crawlin' with midgets!" If I had the muscles of a wheelchair basketball player instead of brittle bones I might have answered, "That's right, Motherfucker. We midgets *are* taking over the world and our first priority is to exterminate big-mouthed assholes like you!"

I didn't, of course, since I can't afford a broken jaw. Usually I just think to myself, "Wait till my friends hear this one!"

As proof that rudeness is not limited to any race or social class, I am reminded of the time a dignified-looking elderly man approached me at intermission in Alice Tully Hall at Lincoln Center. His balding gray head and well-tailored suit projected an air of Ivy League propriety—an impression he promptly blew by saying, "Well, you certainly got the short end of the stick, didn't you?" I swallowed the urge to answer, "Shut up, baldy."

Though I don't like being patronized or pitied, I prefer it to outright mockery or hostility. One day in Woolworth's, a little old lady came up to me and said, "Let you out of the asylum for the day, have they, dear?" All I could do in response was to stifle a laugh and duck down a side aisle. "That's right, lady," I wish I'd said, "I'll see you there later on!"

A related kind of patronizing involves people talking over your head as if you're not sentient: Once, when I was attending college in Birmingham, England, I went to the local post office with two friends. The woman behind the counter looked at Sid and Pete, ignoring me totally, and said, "Taking him out for an airing, are you?" as if I were a piece of laundry. We all collapsed in a heap of laughter once we got out onto the sidewalk.

Patronizing can be more than verbal; it can take the form of unwanted assistance. Once I was sitting at the foot of a flight of steps when two guys appeared and without a word picked me up in my chair and carried me to the top. When I had recovered from my amazement I said, "Excuse me, I know you meant well, but I was only waiting for a friend. Would you please carry me back down now?"

I get around in a large motorized chair, about 150 pounds of hardware. Add my weight and the whole package amounts to more than 200 pounds. Sometimes I have had to argue fiercely with a would-be helper. Some men seem to feel their manhood threatened when I say, "It's much too heavy a load for one person. It takes three or four, at least." When a guy answers, "No problem, I'm strong," I want to say, "Listen, dear, I'm sure you go to the gym, but unless you're an Olympic weight lifter, you'll need some help." As a matter of fact, I have said versions of this a few times, always causing offense, though once in a while I'm wrong in my estimation. Years ago when the elevator in my apartment building broke, two obese-looking guys insisted they could carry me up a flight of stairs. To my surprise, they did the job of four easily. They turned out to be sumo wrestlers!

One real mystery, at least to me, is what makes people associate disability with panhandling or homelessness. I've had coins dropped in an empty coffee cup I was holding, and in one memorable incident, a full cup. One time a nun thrust a fistful of bills at me. "The Lord wants you to have this twenty-five dollars," she insisted. For once I came back with a reply that pleased me: "Who am I to argue with the Lord?" Since I happened to be broke at the time and Sister looked implacable, I took the money. I managed to salve my conscience later on by using some of the cash to buy food for a homeless man.

In another crazy Manhattan encounter, I was wheeling down Broadway minding my own business when a man came up to me and said, "I'd give you a quarter, but since you're so small, I'll give you a dime!" A second man overheard the remark and confronted the first: "What a terrible thing to say to the poor guy. It's bad enough he's a cripple. You don't have to add insult to misery." They went on arguing fiercely, as folks do in New York, so I left them to get on with it and went about my business.

It is natural, I suppose, to be curious about me—I look very different from most people, even from most other people in wheelchairs. We people with osteogenesis tend to physically resemble one another not only in body but also in facial features. We tend to have large heads, deformed and prominent chest bones, large, delicate, and often quite beautiful hands. Because of this similarity in general appearance, I've often been mistaken for someone else. Years ago the movie *Ship of Fools* prompted repeated demands of, "You're Michael Dunn, aren't you?" Later, it was the wondrously talented French Jazz pianist Michel Petrucciani. Coming out of Carnegie Hall once, where I'd just bought tickets for a classical music concert, I was accosted by a woman in a mink coat with, "Oh no, I'm heartbroken! I missed you! I missed your concert!" When I explained that I was merely a relatively unknown poet, she said, "It's wonderful you're a poet, though. I just love poetry!"

I wonder if anyone ever approached Michel Petrucciani and offered, "I love your poetry." I guess I'm just not famous enough for any reciprocal mistaken identity. Being a public person for all the wrong reasons is pretty tiring. If I'm going to be instantly recognizable I would like to be recognized for my own accomplishments, not for someone else's. I certainly don't want to be recognized as the Generic Cripple who gets a quarter splashed in his cup of coffee.

Disability Made Me Do It,
or Modeling for the Cause

Kenny Fries

In 1991, I am living in Provincetown, when I get a phone call from Tom, a local artist. Tom has been hired to do the drawings for an updated version of a well-known guide to gay male sex.

"I want to make sure different types of men are represented in the drawings," he tells me. "I wanted to talk to you about how to best portray a disabled man having sex."

"Don't use a wheelchair to signify the man is disabled," I tell him.

"Where can I find a disabled guy to model for me?" he asks.

"Beats me," I say.

"Would you do it?" There is a pause. "I'll take photos of you having sex and use them as the source for what I'll draw," he explains.

"Sex with whom?" I ask, as I am single for the first time in seven years.

"That's easy," Tom assures me.

Why did I so easily agree to model for the cause?

"I was an understudy in *A Chorus Line*," he tells me as we sit down for what I expect to be a business lunch. "What can you tell me about directing a play in San Francisco?" I was working for a San Francisco theater services organization when I was asked out to lunch by this man who is interested in getting to know his way around the community.

Over salad I tell him what I know about getting a start: classes, the theaters, some people I suggest he call.

After the waiter removes the plates from the table, my lunchmate looks across the table at me and asks, matter of factly: "Do you like to be humiliated?"

17

Even though I know right away what he is talking about, where this conversation is leading, even though no one has ever asked me such a question before, I am intrigued, so I reply, "Why do you ask?"

"Because I know this one guy in Los Angeles who told me that's the only way he can enjoy sex. Pain and humiliation bring up all the times he got attention when he was a kid, so he gets off on it."

For me the operative words in his response are this one guy in Los Angeles. I could answer him by pointing out how many nondisabled men, gay or otherwise, enjoy experiencing sex that way or offer other enlightened responses, but at this moment all I can muster in response is, "Really?"

Two years later, a nondisabled gay male editor who is interested in my work takes me out to lunch at a ritzy New York restaurant.

"I was very interested in the sex in your book," the editor tells me. As I eat I keep nodding encouragement for him to continue.

"I have a cousin who is disabled. We spent a lot of time together growing up in Texas," he says. "My family wasn't very happy about how swishy I was. We lived in oil country and I guess I didn't live up to, well, what they expected a boy to be. My cousin was my only friend. People are very interested in how disabled people have sex, aren't they?"

Puzzled, my first thought is that not many people would be interested in the way I have sex, being that my sexual practices are probably similar to the experiences of most nondisabled gay men. My next unspoken response is: *No, most people aren't interested, but you obviously are.*

Taking into consideration that I might have to work with this well-intentioned man sitting across from me, and that he is paying for this rather expensive lunch, I simply correct his assumption. "Actually, most people do not think of those of us who live with disabilities as sexual at all."

To St. Augustine "beauty was synonymous with geometric form and balance." Regarding human appearance, the Oxford English Dictionary defines handsome as: "having a fine form or figure, usually in conjunction with full size or stateliness." In *Survival of the Prettiest,* psychologist Nancy Etcoff says that throughout history the discourse on beauty is "an aesthetic based on proportion."

When I was young, before we went to sleep, my brother, three-and-a-half years older than I and with whom I shared a trundle bed, teased me about how short I was. "I'm not short," I replied. "Everyone else is tall."

Now, when I wake during the night, I am surprised when I realize my body, lying so closely to Ian's, is of measure. Because above my thighs, my body is of customary length, when lying in bed with him I feel the equality of my body's size. I feel comfortable, at ease, something I do not feel when standing up and talking to someone at a party where I often don't reach anyone's shoulders, or even when sitting down for dinner in a restaurant where usually my feet do not reach the floor. In crowded public elevators I am often unseen, relegated to a back corner where the view is more often the middle of someone's back, or below.

The night before Tom's photo shoot I begin to get nervous. I have not taken off my clothes, been naked, and shared my body with a stranger for many years. How will I feel undressing and getting into bed with someone handpicked for the occasion? How will he react to my disabled legs? I can't sleep. Lying in bed I think about the story of the Thai Queen Number One. Thai kings were polygamous, each queen had a number according to her station. A long time ago, Queen Number One was on her way to visit the king in the ancient capital of Ayutthaya. It was a very hot humid day and Queen Number One decided to stop at the river. As she swam in the river, the Queen's servants watched over her royal possessions. Suddenly, the Queen began to drown. Because no subject was allowed to touch a Queen, number one or otherwise, her servants simply stood and watched her from the shore. She drowned. I wonder if the servants knew Queen Number One was not a good swimmer.

The next morning at Tom's studio he informs me the part of the book that we will model for will be "Biting."

That doesn't sound too heavy, I think to myself, as I introduce myself to George, my partner for the session.

"This should be interesting," I say as I shake his hand. George doesn't seem as nervous as I feel. Is he surprised I am disabled? Did Tom tell him before he agreed? Even though it probably wouldn't have made me any less nervous, I wish I had asked Tom if he had told George about my disability before we met. *Next time remember to ask,* I tell myself, as if this session will be my first step in what is sure to be a nude modeling career.

A few minutes later, Tom leads us up a flight of stairs to the bedroom where the photos will be taken. As Tom sets up his camera, the lights, and other photographic equipment, I sit on the edge of one side of the large double bed; George sits on the other. Slowly, as we small talk over the width of the bed—"How long have you lived in P-town?" "Where do you work?"—we begin to take off our clothes.

I could be chatting with my doctor or making small talk as I undress for a massage. I don't know George well enough, have never seen him until a few minutes ago downstairs—has he ever seen me and my inimitable gait walking down Commercial Street?—to ask if he has ever done this before. What I do know is that he has olive skin, tight curly black hair, dark brown eyes.

"Should we unmake the bed?" George asks.

"Might as well," Tom calls, still busy with his camera.

When George stands up to take the sheet off the bed, I see his unclothed body for the first time. Casually, or trying to appear casual, I take in his hairless chest, the thin trail of darkness that eventually spreads itself around an amply sized penis. I want to look away before I am aroused. I look down at my feet. How much of my body can George see from where he stands on the other side of the bed?

"Why don't you two get to know each other," Tom says as he checks a light he's set up over the bed. And before I can give Tom's suggestion a moment's thought, George has trampolined onto the bed and is pulling me toward him.

Darwin says: "If everyone were cast in the same mould there would be no such thing as beauty."

But here in bed it feels as if the playing field has been literally leveled. Lying in bed with another man, as I am with George, despite my insecurities, I feel more natural. Even though half an hour earlier I did not know him, I am soothed by his fingers grazing my shoulder, the length of my arm.

"Lay on your back," George tells me, and unquestioningly I do so. How often have I done this—getting to know another man first by touch? But this time I'm doing it for the cause, for the accurate representation of people with disabilities, I remind myself as I feel George's lips on the inside of my thigh.

"Nibble him," Tom calls out from behind the camera, and I feel George gently biting my balls.

"That was great," Tom says much too quickly. "I think I've got what I need."

I wish I could say the same thing, I think, reluctantly watching George put back on his clothes.

As we part in the street, I want to ask George not only what the experience was like for him, but specifically what it felt like to touch me, a disabled man. As I often do after having sex, I try to remember if George actually touched my legs. I want to ask him, as I've asked many men after we've first had sex, if we can get together again.

A few days later when I see George in the street, we stop, exchange pleasant small talk, and with my questions still unasked, continue down the street in opposite directions.

Later that week, Tom calls. He wants me to come over to look at the photos, as well as the drawing he has already begun.

When I see the photos and drawing at his studio, I am both surprised and relieved at my reaction. I do not recoil, as I often do when I glimpse myself in a full-length mirror or in a store window as I'm passing by. This time, I recognize the images of myself in both the photos and the drawing as very beautiful. I check within but do not find the usual embarrassment I feel at seeing a representation of my body.

A week later Tom calls. "The art director didn't like it," he tells me. "He said that in the drawing the disability didn't read. He wants me to cut off one of your legs."

"My parents didn't let many well-known doctors do that when I was born," I tell Tom.

"Or I can put in a wheelchair by the side of the bed."

"But that's the easy way out. We talked about this before I agreed to model."

"I know we did."

"What are you going to do?" There is a long pause.

"I can put somebody else's head on your body, then take off one or both of your legs," he offers.

"You can't do that. If you can't use my body as it is you can't use my body at all."

"Now I'm even more behind schedule than I was. I'll have to find another model, reshoot the whole thing, do a whole other drawing," he says before he hangs up the phone.

"The human image has been subjected to all manners of manipulation in an attempt to create an ideal that does not seem to have a human incarnation," writes psychologist Nancy Etcoff.

Months later, when the book is published, no drawing of me is included. Instead, accompanying the section on "Masculinity" is a drawing of a group of otherwise nondisabled men, one fully clothed man sitting in his disability-signifying wheelchair.

As I stare at the drawing, I realize a man with a disability has once again entered the book of myths defined *as* his disability instead of being portrayed as a person *with* a disability. To the large audience who will use this book this might be the only image they might ever see of a disabled gay man. And the message of the drawing: "Despite his having to use a wheelchair, he is a man, too," rather than "Here is a man who also uses a wheelchair."

Leaving the bookstore I am sad at this missed opportunity. Lying in bed that night, I can't get the photos of me and George out of my mind. Did George ever see them? If so, what did he think? "Nibble him." I hear Tom say, as I finally fall asleep.

Waking the next morning, I get out of bed, reluctantly. Who was I kidding? I ask myself as I get up to take a shower. Was modeling for Tom any different from my other brief sexual encounters?

Feeling the strong pulse of the spraying water run over me, it is as if I am back in the showers at the JCC in San Francisco. I hear ancient languages being spoken and closing my eyes the water's heat slowly dissolves the skin of my limbs, then my bones, to wash away time, until I am one of those armless, legless, Greek statues—all torso— something akin to a male Venus de Milo, who despite having no arms or hands, the stump of her upper right arm extending just above her breast, who, despite her scarred face and severed left foot, despite having the big toe cut off her right foot, and a missing left nipple, not being real, is considered one of the most beautiful figures in the world.

Nasty Habits

Bob Guter Interviews Gordon Elkins

Gordon Elkins, businessman and community activist, often doffs his pinstripes for the habit of Sister Anal Receptive, one of The Sisters of Perpetual Indulgence, Inc., celebrated for their charitable (and outrageous) endeavors. Gordon talks to Bob Guter about why he took the veil, how polio influenced his feelings about social activism, and other matters.

BOB: I've been an admirer of The Sisters for years. I'd like to know how you became Sister Anal Receptive.

GORDON: The Sisters came into my life in a roundabout way. Back in 1990 when I had my own company—we did special events productions—I hired someone to work for us who was a walking dream. Pierre was a French Canadian trapeze artist; it was one of those rare situations where our very differences (he was fourteen years younger and had a body to die for) made it possible for us to open different worlds to one another. Somehow I manifested him into my life. I don't know how I did that, but I did. Anyhow, he'd been approached to do some fund-raising events with The Sisters. One involved a gallery opening to celebrate a series of large paintings of all The Sisters by an artist named Thomasina Demaio. Pierre did a trapeze show as part of the opening. Soon after that he became a Sister himself, so I started going to meetings just to spend time with him. Finally one of the founders, Sister Vicious Power Hungry Bitch, said to me, "You attend more of our meetings than our regular members, Gordon. Does this mean you want to join The Sisters?"

BOB: And you were a Sister, just like that?

GORDON: Oh no! It's all very structured. You first become a postulant and then a novice. As it happened. I became a novice at a time when The Sisters' books were in the red. Two of us novices were put in charge of a fund-raising booth at the Folsom Street Fair. To everybody's surprise, we raised $1,100, enough to put The Sisters back in the black. Well, at the very next meeting we were elevated to fully professed members and that same evening I was elected treasurer! At about the same time The Sisters took over Halloween in the Castro. That year we had a gate of about $36,000! I was intent on our being squeaky clean financially, so when I took the books to our accountant he was stupefied, because for the first time every penny was accounted for! I guess that was my road to the presidency, which is where I ended up for a while. That's a *very* short summary of my career as a Sister.

BOB: It's nearly a decade since you met Pierre and took the veil. Two life-altering events?

GORDON: Yes. Lots of changes. Pierre was HIV positive. Back then there were no cocktails, so I pretty much knew what would happen. I took care of him until he died and the time we spent together was magical. Some of it was wild and funny, too. Pierre also performed at the Campus Theater, where he was really, really popular. All of his groupies would wait for him to come out after a show and I'd play the wallflower over by the door. He was good to his fans, but at some point he'd always announce, "Well, I gotta go." Then he'd burst through the doors, I'd hop on the back of his motorcycle and off we'd go into the night, while all the groupies stood there wondering, "Who the hell is *he?!*" Because Pierre was such a talented acrobat (he trained at Le Cirque du Soleil), instead of entering down the aisles like the other performers did he'd balance seat arm to seat arm over people's heads—quite the act. One night when I was sitting way in the back he was crouching over me jerking off to the appreciation of the crowd. What they didn't know was that he was whispering in my ear, "I can't wait to get out of here. These are the cheapest bastards tonight; nobody's tipping. Where are we going to dinner?"

BOB: It sounds like you two were a fabulous team.

GORDON: Oh, you can't imagine! The stuff we did at the theater was incredible. Here's a real secret of the porn stars: Pierre did an act downstairs, too, in what they called the Arena. He had a natural talent for getting everyone involved, with great come-on lines like, "I'm not just here for your pleasure; come down here and pleasure me, too." Of course everybody was too shy to move, so on nights when I was there I was the shill. I'd lean against a pillar across from Pierre and pull it out and start jerking. There I was having an intimate encounter with my own personal porn star in the middle of this public place. Finally he would say, "I'm *not* coming first." Then *I* would climax, everybody else would blow in a great shower, and Pierre and I could get out of there to our dinner or movie.

BOB: There you were, doing this incredible performance sexually, framed by this incredible relationship—was that easy for you to do?

GORDON: The sexual part? I think I was always a closet exhibitionist; Pierre brought that out in me. I've always been an organization junkie, too, so when Pierre brought me into contact with The Sisters he helped me fulfill that other need. When you're shy—and I am, really—organizations, especially "helping" organizations, can be a way to socialize, bypass your wallflower identity. I know that there's a deep connection to my disability, too. I grew up feeling less attractive because of polio. Having something to give made me feel better about myself.

BOB: How has your life been different since Pierre died?

GORDON: For one thing, I haven't really dated anyone since then. I believe that Pierre and I were soul mates. At one point early on I just knew that I would be the one to be with him to the end. Once, not long before he died, he looked at me intently and said, "I don't know why, but in the last couple of weeks I've had so much love for you." We just grew closer and closer. My role was to help him prepare spiritually for his transition, because he was not a spiritual person at all. At one point he talked about suicide, and that always remained an option, but as he got sicker he came to a greater sense of peace. He was accepting at the end. As for me, I discovered what it was like to be with someone in that very spiritual, magical soul mate place where you give and receive without boundaries.

BOB: I know that in the years since Pierre's death your life has changed in other ways, because of post-polio syndrome. Tell me how polio affected your early years, so I can understand what's going on now.

GORDON: I contracted polio six months before the Salk vaccine was available! It was being tested on the East Coast and we lived in the middle of Oklahoma. I was lucky in two ways, though. It affected only my left leg, and because my father had had polio when he was nineteen, my parents knew what they were getting into. I wasn't catered to the way some kids were. I still remember calling my parents to get me something. Their response was, "Get it yourself!" So I'd haul myself into my wheelchair and get what I wanted.

BOB: How did things work out at school?

GORDON: I was able to keep up during regular class time with a two-way radio hookup; after school a teacher came to tutor me for things I couldn't see on the blackboard. I got polio in the fall and was back at school in the spring, in a full leg brace.

BOB: Do you remember how you felt about being separated from your friends? You couldn't go out to play and they could—things like that?

GORDON: I adjusted because my parents never allowed me to think of myself as "handicapped." Also, there'd been such an epidemic of polio in Oklahoma City that I wasn't too unusual. So I guess with some limitations I made friends like everybody else. I wasn't part of the jock crowd, obviously, but I recall *watching* the jocks. There was a boy named Richard Gresham who was on the football team and the wrestling team and God, did I have a crush on him! He had such a body. Before they were stylish he used to wear shorts slit up the side. He'd go out on the football field on his lunch hour to exercise and I'd go watch. I think my being disabled let me watch without it looking strange.

BOB: It sounds as if one "differentness," disability, protected you from being attacked for your other, even more deviant "differentness."

GORDON: That's true. Being disabled was odd enough that I was not suspect for other reasons.

BOB: What was it like for you being gay in high school?

GORDON: I knew I was different but I was still trying to figure out what it meant. I was dating girls, but I never had a "girlfriend." By the time I got to college I was miserable. I knew I was gay but I didn't know what to do with that knowledge. Living in Oklahoma, I thought I was the only one! Fortunately for me, the assistant dean of men took an interest in me and I would study at his place. He was gay—everybody gossiped about him but everybody loved him. He was a savior for me; he validated me because he cared about me. I remember how miserable I was on Saturday nights, but

I think that's when the groundwork was laid for my devotion to volunteer work, the feeling I mentioned earlier about being less self-conscious if you have something to offer. Since I had no social life, I began to get involved in working for my fraternity. To this day they have a Gordon Elkins Service Award. I wonder sometimes if I went back and came out of the closet *there* if they'd still give the award.

BOB: They'd damn well better!

GORDON: Remember, it's still Oklahoma. When I got out of school I worked for a while with a younger fraternity brother. He was interviewing someone for the job of sales director when the subject of "fags" came up. "Well, we don't *have* fags in Oklahoma," he said. "We just line 'em up and shoot 'em." Guess who came out to me not long after that?

BOB: The new sales director.

GORDON: Of course!

BOB: How were you managing physically in the years before the post-polio syndrome hit?

GORDON: Through my freshman year in college I used a full leg brace; I had two pairs of shoes, a black pair and a brown pair— a real fashion statement! When I was younger I had such little usable muscle below the knee that they kept the knee well forward because I had no natural "back knee" control. During college vacation one summer a surgeon cut the bone below my knee, turned my foot around straight again and reattached the bone with a pin. Now I do without the full-leg brace, but I've got to be careful; a dip or a rough spot can send me into an impromptu dance routine—or worse. These days, as my leg is weakening, I know my limitations, but it irritates the hell out of me. Now I walk with a cane and I can't do more than two blocks.

BOB: How do these changes make you feel?

GORDON: At times I feel a lot of anger and frustration, because I have always been so active. And it's tough to know where to put the anger. Sometimes I just have to vent. Slowing down is bad enough, but even scarier is the sense of progressive deterioration. I just know I'm going to end up in a full-leg brace again someday. A lot of the time I'm in denial about it. But you know what? I've discovered that finding ways around the negative stuff is a challenge I can

embrace. Take the Gay Pride Parade, for example. Give it up?
You're out of your mind! Instead of walking I've simply engi-
neered things so that now I ride—in *style!* Being the diva that I am,
that suits me just fine.

Piano Bar

Joel S. Riche

You came by surprise
like a knight to . . .
remember me?
We danced in the crowd
and finally met.
So sweet. So cute.
My heart jumped. I melted as you kissed me
goodnight.
I dreamed of you,
us too . . .
Many possibilities, too much
potential?
My crutches didn't faze you
and you didn't ask Why
What or How.
My heart jumped
as you kissed me.
And I melted.

But I Don't Like You Like That

George Steven Powell

Wish I had a dollar for every time I've heard, "But I don't like you like that" from a guy. Surely by now, at age forty-five, I would be rich enough to support the lifestyle I live, but can't afford. When it came to sucking or fucking, I was just their type, willing and needy. But then, what would you expect if you were born with spina bifida?

Never heard of it? I will spare you the medical jargon: you grow to an adult height of four feet and eleven inches, maybe a little taller if you are lucky and the SB isn't as severe as mine. My misshapen body looks as if someone has taken a rubber mallet and pounded me on the head, thus squashing my upper torso. I have no bowel control whatsoever, because I have no anal sphincter; I've got a urostomy, too, which is an opening in the abdomen that looks like a cherry with a plastic pouch worn over it to collect urine. My atrophied left leg ends in a club foot. The bright side of all this, if there is one, is that I'm not paralyzed, I can walk on my own, and I am sexually functional, which is a blessing and a curse.

Having read that, you can surely see what a kick in the head it was to discover at age five that I was gay (my mother always told me I was "different," she just didn't know *how* different). I honestly thought my attraction for boys was just part of my spina bifida; I had never heard "normal" little boys say anything about liking other boys. To further confuse me, I was brought up in the Church of Christ, which my grandfather founded when my mother's family moved to Henderson, Texas, from Paris, Texas, during the oil boom in 1930.

So the hellfire-and-brimstone preacher in the pulpit pounding his Bible as he spewed scripture had me convinced that God had made me like this because I was a sinner! I left that church when I was eighteen and it took years to free myself of all the guilt. For years I hated God for making me this way and, when I wasn't blaming Him, I was blaming my mother.

Because of all my "special needs," I attended first grade at a private school with three other boys (they were there only because their birthdays fell after September). It's amazing that this school, in a retired teacher's house, existed at all in our little one-horse East Texas town. At recess, the other boys would play army and I would be their nurse, taking full advantage of the situation by making my "wounded soldiers" drop their pants so I could check for broken bones. I never could get them to pull down their briefs, but I got enough of a thrill feeling their crotches, until they pushed my probing fingers away. Guess it scared them when their little pricks got hard from my warm touch.

My favorite part of the day was after recess, when we four boys went to Mrs. Hoover's bathroom to wash up. Little did the kindly, blue-haired lady know what a treat she was giving me! Of course, I could never use the toilet in front of the others for fear they would see my cloth diaper and plastic pants and pouch, but I got an eyeful of their pissing little peckers. I was awed by their ability to urinate on command, the golden liquid streaming from their penises instead of draining from a stoma into a bag like mine. It made my body tingle all over and my little organ hard as a rock. I suppose that experience was the first time I realized just how different I was.

I attended public school after Mrs. Hoover's, but I never used the school rest room the entire eleven years. And, unable to take Phys. Ed., I missed out on watching all my smooth-skinned, preadolescent peers undressing. I began to notice what I was missing in junior high, when I had my very first sexual experience. It was the summer after the sixth grade and I camped out in my playhouse with a cute neighborhood boy my own age. Something told me this was the chance I had been waiting for, so when my naive mother told me to "be careful" because sometimes little boys liked to do "nasty" things, I knew that I had hit pay dirt!

That's when I put my plan into action: I challenged John to a game of Old Maid (of course I had marked the Old Maid card to guarantee my victory). When I lost the first game I told John to "make me do something terrible." He suggested that I walk down to the abandoned pasture behind my house in the dark, alone, which really would have been terrible! I pretended that that was no big deal, as if I did it all the time. John looked surprised as he tried to think of something worse. "Hey, I got it," I piped up. "Make me suck your dick." "Damn, gross,"

John mumbled, yet with a curious glint in his green eyes. "Why the heck would ya wanna do that? Only queers do that shit." I panicked. "You're right, think of something else." "Hmmm, let's see," John said, as his hand slid down his lean, bare chest and concave belly. "Damn, my dick's hard," he murmured with labored breath. "I wanna see it." I knew once John took out his prick I had it made.

He unbuttoned his fly and pulled his cock and balls out above the elastic waistband of his white briefs and, boy, was I surprised! His penis was bigger than my dad's, wreathed with a patch of black hair. I touched it gently, making John flinch. "Suck it," he hissed through clenched teeth, getting up on his knees. I noticed, as I gently began sucking, that it tasted sort of like . . . cauliflower. I wondered what would happen if John came in my mouth. Could I get pregnant? The rest, as they say, is history: John was happy, and I was in love with John.

We continued like this for the rest of the summer, but by the following year, John had found a girl who was free with her favors, so I lost out—only the beginning of many disappointments. The rest of junior high and high school were meaningless, painful, practically sexless years, except for occasionally running across a horny guy on the prowl when he and his girlfriend had broken up. It wasn't only sex I wanted or missed; I wanted to go steady with a guy like the girls did.

After graduating from high school in 1972, I had planned to attend college and major in interior design, for which I had shown a natural talent. But I was so sick of school that I decided to go to work as a freelance window dresser—"visual merchandising" they call it now. For my twenty-first birthday, my sister-in-law took it upon herself to tell my parents that I was gay. My mother cried and I heard my daddy say "God damn" for the first time. Mother announced that she was going to write to the doctor at John Sealy Hospital, where I had had all of my surgeries, and ask him if he could "change" me. What amazed me most about this parental reaction was that I grew up playing with Barbie dolls and going to twirling contests; my room was every little girl's dream: a canopy bed, skirted dressing table, the works. Anyway, when Mama failed to tell me the outcome of her letter, I finally asked her. "He's one too," she said solemnly. "One what?" "What you claim you are." Reluctantly, she went on to tell me that the psychiatrist had informed her that the problem was hers, not mine.

It was now time to leave the nest. I happened upon a quaint two-room guesthouse with a swimming pool behind it. The place had been a beauty shop, appropriately named The Go-Gay Salon (where I once had my hair frosted, by the way). I was having a blast, a genuine social life, meeting all sorts of men. One new friend and I became a team, using him for bait when we went to rest areas and parks seeking sexual partners. When we found someone we liked, he would fuck him and I would suck him—a match made in heaven.

This new friend also introduced me to a very special fifteen-year-old boy, another John, someone I had been eyeing ever since he'd turned from a cute kid into a handsome young man. My friend brought John over one night and we had a three-way. John's tennis-player body was so hot! He was willing to please, nothing bothered him, and he started dropping by on his way home from school when he felt the "urge," which was often. John was the first guy that I rimmed. I had never seen a guy's asshole before and I was fascinated with the tiny pink orifice, how it expanded and contracted when I swirled the tip of my tongue across it. I saw then what an asset (excuse the pun) it was to have one and just what I was missing!

I fell madly in love with John Number Two, once again mistaking sexual gratification for love. It was during this period that I went to my first gay bar, where I found myself right back where I'd started, a gay world filled with gorgeous guys and vicious queens. Most of my school classmates had grown up with me and were used to my disability, but here, in a world where you were ridiculed for wearing last season's Ralph Lauren, nobody knew me. I had to reinvent myself, I had to protect myself by becoming wittier and sharper than those wicked, forked-tongued monsters. That's when I discovered the courage builder of all courage builders—alcohol: that magic elixir, mixed with some joints and a little speed, transformed me from a mild-mannered, sweet person into a queen bitch.

After three drinks, I could rip someone apart at fifty paces, reduce him to tears! And the more I drank the meaner I became. The crowd loved me; they really loved me! Over time, it took more and more alcohol to get me to the desired state of total bitchiness (my exits grew a lot less glamorous than my entrances). The alcohol gave me the courage for something I had wanted to try ever since I saw a show in Dallas, Texas—drag. When even drinking began to lose its power, I learned to medicate with things. Every time I got depressed (almost daily) I went out and bought another antique or painting or knick-knack, filling my tiny place with wall-to-wall furniture, covering every surface with more useless objets d'art.

Did it make me any happier or solve my problems? Of course not. It only made me feel good in the moment and propelled me sky-high into debt. Stress from overwork and staying out all night drinking began to affect my health. Still, with everything I had accomplished—or thought I had—I hated myself more than ever. My list of sexual encounters had reached about thirty, but none of them cared anything about me, and I was still afraid to let anyone see me naked.

Oh, a few were interested in more than a blow job and I did have anal intercourse with two of them. Mind you, it was in the pitch dark, I was wearing a robe, and drunk out of my mind! By the way, one good thing about not having an anal sphincter: no pain at penetration. I would be slurring, "Is it in yet?" after the guy had already ejaculated! Even if I'd shit all over them, no matter—I wouldn't remember the next day. God created blackouts for a reason. But all the money and all the things in the world couldn't buy what I really wanted: a man to love me. Every time I got the nerve to tell my latest trick that I loved him, I would once again hear, "I like you, a lot, but not like that."

By Christmas 1981, my drinking was completely out of hand. It was ruining my work and friends no longer wanted me at their parties. Once again, right back where I started: no friends, no lovers. So, I did what any self-respecting queen would do: sobered up, and only then checked myself into the nut ward of a hospital in Tyler, Texas, thirty-five miles from home. I couldn't dare check in drunk, although that's what I was there for! I didn't have shock treatments, or much real treatment of any kind, just a bunch of tests to determine if all that alcohol had damaged my brain or vital organs. So, with a salve and a shove and a prescription for Antabuse—a drug that makes you wish you were dead if you drink alcohol—I was released from the hospital, figuring my new life would change everything, even my chances of finding true love.

Wrong. All that had changed was that I was sober now. Still, they say you have to change one thing—everything—if you want to stay sober, and I did. I started by weeding out friends who didn't support my sobriety. I threw myself into my work, taking on even more clients than before. I moved home with my parents (huge mistake). I was thoroughly miserable.

I saw John Number Two a few times, but he wouldn't come over to my parents' house because they knew his family. About a year later, John got married and I was devastated. Again the stress of work and life in general landed me back in the hospital, this time with a kidney infection. When I got out this time I sold my wallpaper and fabric samples (big investments for a decorator) and went to work for someone else. That didn't work, either. I ended up back in the hospital in December 1983 with an even more serious kidney infection. My urologist told me if I didn't quit work I was going to kill myself.

I went on permanent disability in 1984. I felt lousy about that, as if I had given up, and I guess in many ways I had. Flat broke, except for Social Security, I began medicating my deep depression with food. I ballooned from 115 pounds to 150. My hair started falling out. It was all over but the crying—which I did my share of. I never even left my parents' house and saw only the few friends who would still have anything to do with me.

By 1985 I knew I had to make a change, so I moved out on my own again. Since I still had all my "things" I was able to put together a nice place. A lot of good that did, though, because the old gang wasn't around anymore. I floated through the remainder of that decade in a sober haze as friends died all around me. I vowed never to have sex again, as if I were really giving up something! But, in April 1989, John Number Two called to tell me he was now divorced and had moved back to Henderson. So much for vows. I never really put much faith in them anyway.

I was nervous as a cat—smoking one cigarette after another—the morning John called and wanted to drop by. He was about thirty now and, if possible, looked even better than the last time I had seen him. Of course, I knew what he wanted and was glad to oblige, except for the AIDS thing. I knew I was fine, but hadn't a clue about John. After a brief tour of my new place he was ready for old times in bed. I did one of the most difficult things I had ever done; I had the "AIDS talk" with him. As I suspected, John was insulted that I would even insinuate that he had "it," but admitted that he had never been tested. "So," John began, sitting on the side of my bed, "this means no more blow jobs, huh?" I took a deep breath. "Not as you knew them, no."

John lay on my bed and peeled down his jeans and white briefs and I positioned myself between his long legs. All I could see when I took hold of his rigid cock was the word "death." I wasn't prepared for this. For openers, neither of us had a condom. So, with my thumb covering his piss-slit, I cautiously licked his thick shaft and furry balls; eventually I got him off with a hand job. He wasn't a happy camper and I haven't seen him since.

I knew I didn't want to decorate anymore because I was sick and tired of dealing with rich, spoiled, neurotic clients. Out of the blue, I decided to try my hand at writing. My friends laughed at me. One of them, who'd been a journalism major at Baylor University, told me that I didn't understand the art of writing, but he also gave me the best advice anyone could have: "Put sex in your stories and they'll sell." He was right.

After my many attempts at writing "literature" were met with nothing but rejection slips, I threw in the proverbial towel and decided to try my hand at "dirty stories." I had read lots of second-rate steamy stories, so I knew that I had to do better, but what could I write about? My pathetic sexual experiences would never sell. Voila! The ultimate fantasy world. For once in my life I could be anyone I wanted—a tall, hunky, blond with a huge cock—anybody. I could graft my fantasies on the people and places I really did know, such as those gorgeous cowboys I'd see driving around town in their butch trucks. Why not make them gay?

Despite more rejections, I kept banging away on my ancient electric typewriter, just knowing that the cops were going to burst through the door and arrest me for all the filth I was composing! Finally, in 1993, I received not an acceptance, but very encouraging words from a female editor who said if I changed a few things—made my story hotter, took out the golden shower scene because it wouldn't pass the Canadian censors—that she would like to have a second look at it. I worked all night long on that story and mailed it back the very next day.

About two weeks later, the day after Thanksgiving, I received my first contract. I couldn't believe it! I had never been so excited over making a measly hundred bucks in my life. And the true beauty of all this was that the editor had no idea about my disability, my age, nothing—zip. For once, I had been judged solely on my work and my work alone. Oh, what a feeling!

I wrote another and sold it. Then another and another. It seemed as if everything I wrote was golden! One day the magical spell broke and I opened an envelope with the dread rejection slip. I cried. I cursed. How could God do this to me? I had adjusted to the fact that I would never find the love of my life, but to take away my fantasies, too? After a day or so of this pity party I pulled myself together and dug the typewriter out of the trash. (I had sworn to never write again. Talk about dramatic!)

I decided that maybe that particular editor had tired of my stories, so I wrote a humdinger, sent it off to *Advocate Men,* and it sold. By now, my cynical friends were scratching their heads with amazement, as was I, but puzzled or not I was confident enough to start sending my stories to many different gay magazines, selling a story to every single one of them! They loved me; they really loved me!

Frequently asked questions: "Do I ever get off while writing these stories?" Yes, but believe it or not, writing about sex can be boring. "Where do you come up with all these ideas?" Everywhere. A simple everyday occurrence can turn into a sex free-for-all. "Are your characters based on guys you have had sex with and your own experiences?" A few, loosely. "Do your stories ever have characters with disabilities?" Only one that's sold. The protagonist had a urostomy like me. It was published a few years back in *First Hand* magazine, titled, "Things Aren't Always What They Seem." I've learned that disabled characters aren't popular in porn mags. When they are allowed, the disability has to involve arms or legs, never torsos or genitals, God forbid. I was shocked that the one I wrote was published. "Do you use your real name?" Never!

Ever since a friend gave me his old Mac last January and I got on the Internet, my writing has slowed down quite a bit. I am taking a break as I discover the joys of meeting other gay men, especially men with disabilities.

And, yes, I am still looking for the love of my life, someone who will say, "Hell, yeah, I like you like that. I love ya; I really love ya!"

Working It Out

Steven Sickles

When I was in high school, before Donna Summer even had a record deal, my friends and I wandered through our lives reading, writing, and painting to the sounds of Donovan and Leonard Cohen. We were longhaired intellectuals. Fearless and buoyed by our own self-righteousness, we fought to maneuver funds from new gymnasium equipment to improve our pathetic library collection. We were loathed by our peers and befriended by our teachers.

The idea of training with weights was laughable. What a waste of time! How self-indulgent and narcissistic could you be? Besides, the results were monstrous. And, of course, everyone believed that one day those gorgeous bulges would deflate to messy masses of fat.

Many years later, after a bout with hepatitis B, I was alarmingly thin and yellow. I was finished pretending I wanted anyone other than another man in my arms at night. And, yes, I could finally admit it— I love muscles! Who, after all, did I think I was kidding for all those years? I was the kid who would swipe Charles Atlas advertisements from the back pages of *Esquire* magazine while waiting for a haircut, to squirrel away in my closet. Later, under the sheets, I would drool over their ragged edges, a flashlight ruining all that expensive dentistry in an attempt to keep *both* hands free. A confusing concoction of envy and lust for an adolescent boy.

But how was I going to ensnare a beefy boy with my skinny ass? If I wanted a man with muscles, I reasoned, I'd have to get some of my own. As a fat adolescent, I had tried to curb my appetite and do some weight training just to keep from going completely to hell. The dusty reminders of my lack of discipline still lay in my parents' basement. But this was different. This was going to be my last chance. I was all of twenty-eight years old. If I did not stick to it this time, I would be hopelessly out of shape, forever, capable of attracting only myopic octogenarians, never to know the thrill of rock hard flesh against my own.

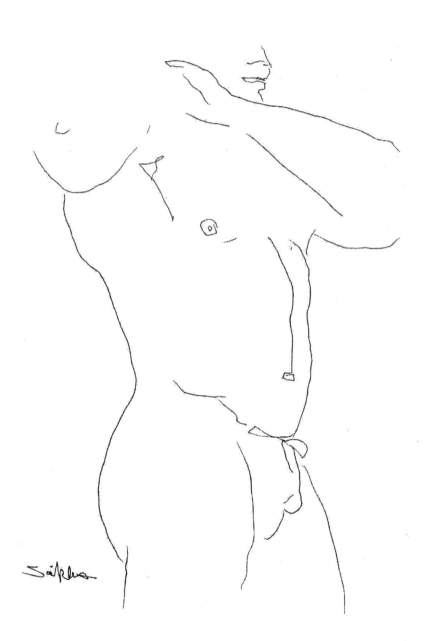

So I marched down to Fourteenth Street in New York City to buy two twenty-five-pound dumbbells. I tossed them around in my Chelsea studio apartment, imagining I was giving Arnold a run for the money.

From these humble beginnings I found I could train regularly. More important, once others noticed, my passion was confirmed. Several years later, after abandoning my insecurity about joining a gym and becoming a regular at Gold's, I was obsessed, confident, and proud of my new physique. I wasn't going to win the Mr. America title, but I could appear in a bikini without embarrassment. Self-indulgent? Narcissistic? Sure. But, I reasoned, it was like working on a sculpture that would never be done, a work in progress. Besides, I had always been timid and insecure. Now, I was self-assured. Vain, surely, but not conceited or arrogant. I had never thrown a punch in my life, but at least now I looked as though it might hurt if I did. This was good.

Then, on February 23, 1996, I became ill with meningitis and the world I had fashioned started to unravel. Complications from the disease caused my blood to clot. Two occlusions settled in the arteries leading to my right hand. In the weeks following my hospital stay, I was weak, pathetically thin, scarred, chemically dependent, and unable to sleep—but I was alive. And there was more. The clots were gone, but over the next two months the fingers on my right hand curled and blackened like charred wood. Gangrene. In May they had to go. I was now living proof of the hazard of placing too much value in personal appearance. My elegant hand, a marvel of design and function, had been replaced with a blunt spade.

Today, this pathetic appendage resembles a sightless desert mole, but it once was as gruesome as something out of a Vincent Price movie. It's amazing to me, looking back, that I agreed to have the nasty thing photographed before the amputation.

My friend, Mark I. Chester, runs a Tuesday evening gay men's sketch group. For years I have been both a model and one of the artists. Mark is a fine photographer, whose idiom is anything left of center. His sexually charged photographs are at once alarming and provocative. He approached me about the possibility of documenting in black and white what had happened to me. Incredibly, I said yes. Often misinterpreted, the photographs that resulted are viewed by some as an objectification. Critics are repulsed by what they see as my blatant exploitation. To my mind, the value of documentary photography depends heavily on context and intention, so these pictures seem no more exploitative than the *Life* photographs of war-torn Vietnam or photos by Diane Arbus. But it's not my point here to defend them. What's more intriguing to me is my view of the whole process, *then,* and my reaction to seeing the photographs, *now.*

During the shoot, I was mystified by Mark's regular departures to compose himself. My feelings of denial were so strong that I couldn't imagine he could be so moved by what he saw. I tried to remain affable and cheerful, my vanity and cooperative spirit overpowering any thought of how I would ultimately react to seeing a frank reflection of how I appeared to the rest of the world.

To this day, I am unable to look at any of those pictures, except those in which my right hand is obscured. In fact, any picture taken before my illness or since that includes a view of my hands, is difficult for me to look at. None is on display anywhere in my house or office. Although my hand is healed, I avoid looking at it, even in a mirror. Pictures taken prior to 1996 fill me with a sense of longing and loss. The pictures taken by Mark are, for me, the stuff that nightmares are made of. Current pictures are difficult to look at, like bravely smiling images of a friend or relative who has died. My eye is drawn to the hands. I never see anything else.

So what do I do, now that I feel well again? In the days following my release from the hospital, I was pleased to be alive and breathing fresh air. But as I recovered more of my life the way I remembered it, I realized it could never be as it was. What was I going to do, now that it appeared I would be unable to train as I once did? I had put too much stock in the way I looked to toss all that aside simply because it might now be even harder to do.

After three months (and twenty pounds) I went back to the gym to see if I could reverse the direction my saggy butt was heading in. I was, after all, still vain, gay, and single. Surprisingly, there were many exercises I could manage, given what was left of my right hand and the fact that, even after the amputation, I still had a wrist. After several designs and many months, my prosthetist and I came up with a device that helped me to pull weights toward me, thus allowing me to increase the poundage and number of repetitions for each exercise, and to train all body parts again.

Okay, I can't do just what I did in January 1996. I will certainly never enter a physique competition. And I will forever look with envy at the big boys in the gym. For me, the value now is in the trying. The standard isn't the same, but the point is identical. The push to see what I can accomplish, how I can mold myself with stubborn determination, hasn't changed.

Two years later, I still shy away from photographers. But when I put on my rubber hand and a pair of worn jeans and walk around the streets of San Francisco, I can still turn the heads of handsome men. It's probably the body I refuse to let grow old gracefully, but it could be the goatee. I'm keeping both, just in case.

When I lost all the digits from my right hand to meningitis, I feared I might have lost some other things as well, things I considered integral parts of myself, such as the ability to draw and paint. My first attempts were weak artistically and crippling emotionally. What I have discovered is that I draw as well with my left hand as I ever did with my right. But what I also realize is that when I draw or paint, it is the only time I completely forget about what I've lost.

Boy Scout of America

Robert I. Roth

As the pink Oldsmobile headed north on the Sunshine State Turnpike, its chrome gleamed in the Florida sun. In the passenger seat, I looked at the map, giving my dad directions in a loud voice on how to get to Sebring. At ten years old, I was excited to be off on my first experience away from home to spend a week with other Boy Scouts from all over the state.

In the backseat were two boys, Denny and Charlie. Denny was from the North Miami troop that I belonged to; Charlie was a friend of Denny's from another troop. I knew in some indistinct way that I was different from Denny and Charlie: I wanted to be their friend, to be liked. I knew they were hearing and I wasn't.

I was taught, however, at school and at home, that being deaf didn't make a difference. Though I had hearing friends in my neighborhood, I never thought of them that way. They were just kids on my block. I went to school on a small bus with other kids who were deaf, blind, or disabled. The yellowness of the bus screamed out, "There's something wrong with the kids in this bus! Come and look!" I was ashamed that I didn't go to my neighborhood school, only two blocks away. At my school, among the kids who moved their hands in a combination of sign and voice, I had many friends. Confronted with the occupants in the backseat, I hadn't the slightest idea of how to befriend boys who could hear.

In between looking at the map and watching for the road signs to make sure we were going in the right direction, I would study the boys in the backseat. They were visibly talking: their jaws were moving up and down, punctuated by what looked like giggling or laughing. I marveled at their familiarity with each other: hands lightly poking Denny's thighs to point out some happening in a passing car, or elbows nudging Charlie's chest, provoking laughter at an unheard joke. Their loud laughing my hearing aid could pick up; it was their conversation I couldn't understand. My dad was too busy driving to repeat what was being said. (My mother always repeated everyone's conversations to me at family gatherings; she became famous for her loud voice.)

I desperately wanted to know what the two boys were talking about. I had long ago mastered the art (or had I?) of pretending to understand what was going on, by laughing at the right moments. I always made sure that I looked as though I was listening, and I laughed when others laughed. The secret was to have the beginnings of a laugh on your face. It may appear like a perpetual grin, but at the right time, it could be interpreted by others as a laugh. This took care of that split-second between the time that others laughed and the moment when you realized that yes, true to business, they were laughing. So, pretending to understand Denny and Charlie, I was laughing away without the slightest clue as to what I was laughing about. It often seemed, from their curious glances at me and each other, that they didn't have a clue as to what I was laughing about either.

In between figuring out what the boys were saying and looking at the map, I focused on the rocket ship perched on the car's broad hood. Or I counted off the white stripes on the road that the rocket seemed to be whooshing over. After several hours of counting white stripes, we finally arrived at Sebring.

Dad dropped us and our backpacks off at the main building. My sense of adventure overcame the momentary terror of seeing the Eighty-Eight drive off, its tires spewing a trail of dust. I didn't know anyone except Charlie and Denny, and they didn't really count.

A man seeming years older than Dad walked up to the three of us; he had the look of authority about him. He talked with the two boys; they started following him, so I did too.

After several attempts at conversing with me, the man pointed to some tents grouped around a clearing and tried to tell me that I should go there, as if I should pick a tent and get settled in.

I chose a tent in one corner because it seemed empty. Inside were two canvas cots. I laid out my sleeping bag and got out the *Mad* magazine I'd bought the previous day. I still remember the cover clearly; it had the numbers "1961" printed boldly across the cover along with the words, "The most upside-down year since 1881!" Turning the magazine upside down confirmed that the numbers still read "1961." I felt upside down, too. What was I doing at Sebring? Who was going to talk to me here? No one waved their hands to talk. Those who did try to talk with me curtly waved me away whenever I responded with a "What?"

I remember little of that week. Nothing made sense to me; nothing was explained to me. I figured out the activities by following along with whatever anyone else was doing. The first night, I followed the others to an odd building with no roof; upon entering I discovered it was a communal shower.

I was horrified at the thought of taking my clothes off in front of other people; no one had prepared me for something so unthinkable. I walked out and went a week without taking a shower, preferring instead to sponge myself at the washbasins near the latrines. Otherwise, the week was a blur of obtaining badges for cooking, canoeing, whittling, and so forth. These badges were for a pea green sash that was part of the Scout uniform.

I don't remember how Robert and Brad, the two Eagle Scouts, knew that I was lonely. I had seen them before during the week; they always seemed to be together. I had wanted to befriend Robert, but with Brad always around, there never was an opportunity. Robert was the taller of the two, with broader shoulders. His hair was black, cut longer than the crew cut that Brad and other boys had. The fact that Robert and I shared the same name appealed to me—we had something in common. Surely, I thought, he would like me and be a friend if I could somehow meet him.

I remember walking back to my tent alone when Robert and Brad caught up with me. Robert asked how I was getting along. Surprised at their sudden interest in me, I said, "Fine"—my usual denial when there was a problem related to my not being able to hear.

Then they suggested a prescription for making friends; it was used by world leaders and immediately bonded people together. Did I want to know that secret to making friends? I was so lonely and desperate to have friends in this place miles away from home that I was game for anything.

Robert described to me the secret, while Brad nodded in assent. The secret was to get on your knees and take the other person's penis into your mouth and blow it. I was surprised; like the communal shower, no one had ever told me about "blowing." Brad, seeing the look of incredulity on my face, followed Robert's lead and picked up on the world leader story: "That's how President Kennedy and Premier Khrushchev get along. It's done all over the world." Well, that seemed like irrefutable evidence to a ten-year-old mind. It took a few more minutes for them to overcome whatever doubts I had left.

They led me to their tent, which of course looked just like mine, but without my things in it, their tent lacked the security mine had.

Robert told Brad to go first while he stood lookout in front of the tent. I continued standing, at a loss what to do. It was Robert I wanted to be friends with.

I looked up at Brad's face. He seemed to stand at least two feet taller than me. He motioned for me to kneel.

I hesitated, not sure of what he had said.

His hand moved to my shoulder and insistently pushed me down.

I bent down on the dirt floor. I felt a burning in my cheeks. I faced his belt buckle emblazoned with the words "Boy Scouts of America." His hands blocked my vision as they fumbled with the buckle. Then the zipper glided down, revealing his white underpants, their brightness in contrast to his dark green pants.

As his hands pushed down both underwear and pants to his knees, I was intrigued by the downy hair just below his navel. Then I saw his penis. It was odd, different, and larger than mine, surrounded by smallish hairs. I'd never seen another penis before, aside from my brother's when we took baths together.

Brad pushed his penis against my lips. I was surprised by its soft, silky texture. I didn't know what to do, but I felt a growing sense of confusion. I realized that I shouldn't be here, yet my body remained fixed, unable to move. I felt, again, harder, his hand on my shoulder. Looking up at his face, he broke his leer to tell me to just blow on it.

Fingers from his other hand seemed to pry my mouth open. His penis went into my mouth. Oddly, it grew firmer and hotter inside. The heat of its skin felt strange and, for some nameless reason, comforting. I blew on it, as instructed, inhaling and exhaling through my nose. I willed myself not to touch the penis with my tongue.

After a few minutes of steady blowing, Robert came inside the tent. Brad released me while Robert took his place. Robert's pants were already down around his knees; his penis was already hard.

I felt defeated. I finally understood that Robert's intentions were not friendly.

My mouth accepted Robert, as it had Brad. I felt Robert's hands at the back of my head. They were insistent, pushing my head forward. My tongue inadvertently touched his penis, reveling at its smooth texture. My saliva wet the bottom of his penis. A sudden release of pressure, coupled with the natural tendency to pull back, slid my mouth backward over his penis.

This was followed once again by pressure moving my head toward his body. As my nose nestled momentarily in his sparse hair, the light aroma of sweat made me dizzy. As Robert held my head firmly, I continued this motion for what seemed an eternity.

Then Robert stopped, pulling out of my mouth.

I looked up.

Robert told me to go, waving me out. I got up and pulled aside the tent's flap, surprised at the sudden sunlight. No one was out there.

I walked toward my tent. Inside, I tried to figure out what had happened. This hadn't made any friends for me—what had I done? In a panic of regret, I grabbed my drinking glass and ran out of the tent toward the washbasins.

At one of the sinks I filled up my glass and rinsed my mouth. Did I do that? I rinsed again. Why don't they like me? I rinsed again and again.

The day came to leave camp. I was glad to see Charlie's dad. He said, "Hello," the first nice word anyone had said to me in the last few days. When Denny and Charlie backed away from me and were only too happy to let me sit in the front seat of the red Chevrolet, I realized that the whole camp knew what had happened.

I felt my face burn.

But I consoled myself with the thought that my dad's car was a year newer and an Oldsmobile . . .

A few months later, I came home from school and picked up the mail on the way into the house. My heart raced as I noticed the "Boy Scouts of America" logo on the envelope, and it was addressed to my dad.

I had not gone to a troop meeting since camp ended, refusing to go whenever my mother suggested it. I was sure that Denny had told the whole troop what happened. Fear ran through my body; my secret was known to all the scoutmasters and now my father would be informed of the sordid truth! He would be totally disgusted with me and never look at me again.

I went into my bedroom, locked the door, and stared at the envelope. With trepidation, I opened it and read the letter. The top of the paper announced in small letters, "Founded 1908 by Sir Robert Baden-Powell."

Fear, relief, and revulsion went through my body as I read these words: "Your son recently had the time of his life Scouting at Boy Scout Camp in Sebring, Florida. A contribution to continue the work of the Boy Scouts of America would be appreciated so that other boys may also enjoy scouting."

I tore up the letter into small pieces and threw it away.

Rolling On
(from Chapter 3)

Carmelo Gonzalez

At the age of thirteen, Carmelo Gonzalez underwent surgery to correct complications caused by cerebral palsy. This chapter of his autobiography begins when Carmelo returns home after three months of rehabilitation, already dreading the turmoil he knows he'll find there.

When I got home, everybody came to see me, but I still wanted to be back in the hospital. My mother had moved to a three-room apartment in Richmond Hills, Queens, where I slept in the living room, and my mother and Ralph (my stepfather) slept in the bedroom. They told me that the bedroom was mine, but I had to stay in the living room until they got a sofa bed. It took three years for us to get one, but we finally fixed the room up the way I wanted it. I helped them paint it light blue. While we were painting we had a paint fight. We had a lot of fun painting that room.

When my mother told my father that I was home again, he wrote and asked her to let my brother Nelson and my sister Carmen take me to see him in prison. Whenever he had visitors, my father would ask them to bring some drugs in a balloon. The reason you use a balloon is so the prisoner can swallow it, then shit it out and clean it. We hid the balloon in my wheelchair, where they couldn't really check.

My father gave me a hug and we talked until it was safe, then he took the balloon and swallowed it. He told me that he'd made me a picture. I had to wait until we left to get it. It was a picture of a boy with three puppies jumping on him. I hung it on the wall at home and whenever I looked at it I would think about my father. I wish that I still had that picture.

To get home we had to walk fifteen blocks to the train station. On the way, Nelson wanted to scare me so he started running with me. He was zigzagging and tried to run Carmen down with the wheelchair. At first I liked it, but then he started going too fast. I was getting scared so I told him to stop. He called me a chicken.

Everything was good for a month or so, until New Year's Eve, when we had a party. Everyone was drinking, but I didn't want any. I hate alcohol. I hated the way my family would act when they got drunk. They would always get into a fight and New Year's Eve was no exception. Everything was fine until one in the morning, and then the shit hit the fan. I don't remember how it began, but Irene and my mother started arguing and Nelson got into it. Then Ralph got into it. Before you knew it everyone was fighting.

Nelson got mad and locked himself in the bathroom. I was going crazy. I wanted to walk out of the house but I couldn't so I sat on my bed watching everybody fight like cats and dogs. When Irene saw Nelson leaving she tried to go after him. My mother blocked the door, so Irene ended up climbing out the window. Imagine a woman ready to give birth at any minute climbing out of a first-floor window.

The fight seemed to last forever. Everybody went home, but my mother and Ralph kept on fighting until daylight. Ralph picked up the coffee table and smashed it on the floor. I was crying and trying to tell them to stop. They kept on fighting until my mother locked herself in the bathroom because she was afraid that Ralph was going to hit her. Sometimes when he did hit her, she would hit him back or scratch him. I couldn't do anything but watch what was going on.

My mother is an epileptic and she would sometimes have seizures when they were fighting. It would scare the shit out of me then because I thought she was going to die. Once she stopped drinking, the seizures diminished. You don't know how much I thank God that she stopped drinking. When she would drink, she would turn into a . . . I don't know what to call it. It was like someone would take over her body. I don't know what, but it wasn't my mother.

When I couldn't take my mother and Ralph fighting anymore I would think about killing myself. Sometimes when they went to sleep or went out, I would go into the kitchen to get a knife and try to stab myself, or go into the bathroom and get some pills. I never had the guts to do it. I wished that I could walk so I could run away. Sometimes I would picture myself going down the stairs in my wheelchair. I wished that someone would kidnap me; that's how much I wanted to leave. Since I couldn't, I had to sit there and hope that they would get tired and take their asses to bed so I could go to sleep myself. Before I would go to bed, I would take whatever they had left and pour it down the sink.

There were times when I would only have three or four hours of sleep, but no matter how tired I was I would always want to go to school, just to get out of that house. All the other kids liked Fridays and hated Mondays. It was the opposite for me. I think I was the only kid that hated three-day weekends and vacations, because they meant that I had to stay home and hear people fighting. I never wanted to miss school. It was the only place where I got away for a few hours, so I never wanted to miss even one day.

Do you know how it feels when you want to get out of your house, and you can't? It's like dying of thirst and there is a cup of water five feet away, but you can't get the water because you are tied down in a chair. Then imagine that you have to sit there and watch other people drinking it. That's how I felt looking out the window, watching the kids in my neighborhood playing outside.

Derek and Nicholas, two guys in my class, went to a club together every other Saturday. It was like a boys and girls club for handicapped kids. I knew that I needed to get into the club, so I asked them how. Derek didn't want to tell me, but Nicholas gave me the phone number. I had no idea how much that place was going to change my life. I had somewhere to go every other Saturday from nine in the morning until six at night. I could be out of the house when my mother and Ralph started to drink. There were a lot of things to do there. You could play sports, do arts and crafts, or just make new friends.

One day I met a man named Jeff who worked there. He was disabled too, but not that much. He was small and used a wheelchair. We didn't know what was wrong with him so we called him a midget. He would always talk to me. I liked having someone to talk to. I thought he was a nice guy. I got to like him, until one day he asked, "Do you like boys?" I couldn't believe what I heard.

"WHAT! What did you say?"

"Do you like boys?"

"Why are you asking me that?" I asked him.

He put his hand on my shoulder and said, "I watch you and I see how you look at them."

"What are you talking about? I look at them like I look at everybody else."

He just patted me on the leg and told me that he understood. I knew that I had some feelings for boys, but I didn't know why I was having them. I thought I was crazy for having those feelings, so I learned how to deny them and hide them. I wasn't until years later that I could admit to myself that I was gay.

I thought Jeff was the only one I could trust until one Saturday. The heat wasn't working, so we had to keep our coats on. I had to go to the bathroom, but I couldn't go with my coat on. He said he could help me if I wanted him to.

He told me that the bathroom for us kids wasn't working, but there was another bathroom we could go to. I didn't think anything of it, so we went up to the next floor. When we got there it was very small, only one wheelchair would fit. He told me to go in with my wheelchair and he would get out of his and walk in. After using the bathroom, I started to pull up my pants. He told me that he would help me pull up my pants, but he pulled down his own pants instead.

"What are you doing?" I asked him as I tried to get up.

He pushed me back down and told me, "Sit down and don't move."

He tried to grab my penis. I pushed his hand away and said, "Leave me alone! I want to get up."

He told me to shut up and sit still. I went to try to open the door to get out and started to cry.

"Shut up," he said. "You know you like it, so shut up or I'll hit you."

He grabbed my penis and he told me to hold his. I tried to pull my hand away, but he was holding my hand too tight. The more I tried to pull away, the tighter his grip got. I realized that I couldn't do anything but stay still and let him do what he wanted.

He asked if I liked what he was doing to me. I told him No. It felt to me like I had to go to the bathroom again. I didn't know what was happening to me.

"Stop, I have to go to the bathroom. I'm going to go on myself!" Just then, I came. I got scared. That was the first time that I had ever ejaculated. After I came, he made himself come on me. I was really scared and didn't know what he was going to do next.

After it was over he grabbed me by my neck and said, "You better not tell anybody what happened here, because it was your fault. You made me do this. If you do tell anybody they are not going to believe you, and I will kill you. I know your address. I will go to your house and kill you and your family."

He grabbed my neck even harder. I really thought that he was going to kill me. We heard someone coming so he let me go and pulled up his pants. He took some toilet paper and wiped up the sperm and pulled my pants up. Just before he went to open the door he told me, "Remember, if you ever tell anybody what happened, I'll kill you."

I really thought he might kill me. He made me feel it was all my fault. When I went back downstairs I stayed in a corner by myself and started to cry.

A counselor saw me and asked, "What's wrong, Carmelo? Are you all right?"

I told her my stomach hurt. Jeff came up to us and asked what was going on. She told him that I was having stomach pains. Then she asked me if I wanted to lie down. I said Yes, thinking I would get away from Jeff. As we were leaving, someone came and told her she was needed. Jeff said he would take care of me.

He pulled me to the side, grabbed my arm real hard and said to me, "I hope you wasn't thinking about telling her what we did!"

"No, I wasn't! Let my arm go, you're hurting me."

"Good! Don't forget what I told you. I will kill you and your family. I have your address." He showed me that he did have my address. "Anyway, nobody is going to believe you."

The next Saturday I tried to stay away from him, but he got me alone again, this time in the elevator.

"How is my special friend doing?" he asked me.

I didn't say anything. I just looked down.

"What's wrong? Look at me," he said as he pulled my head up. When he reached to stop the elevator I knew he was going to molest me again.

"It's been two weeks since I saw you. I missed you. Did you miss me?" he asked me.

I didn't say anything. I just looked back down. When I saw his hands going toward my pants I tried to stop him, but he grabbed my hand and said, "Don't fight me, Carmelo. You know you like it."

I was afraid that he was going to hurt me so I didn't do anything to stop him. He opened my pants and grabbed me and started to jerk me off, then he opened his pants. The bell rang to let him know that someone needed the elevator. At first he didn't stop, but they kept on ringing, so he had to stop.

"Remember, Carmelo. Don't tell anybody about this, or I'll kill you."

After that, there were nights when I couldn't sleep. Every time I closed my eyes I would see Jeff doing what he did to me. He started to call to ask if I told anyone. Then he would talk dirty to me. He would ask me if I ever had anybody put their dick up my ass, and he would tell me that he wanted to do it to me. He said he wanted to show me how it feels to get it in the ass. Before he hung up, he would always remind me that if I ever told anybody what happened, he would kill me. He told me that what had happened was because I wanted it to, that it was my fault, and if I told anyone they would think I was making it up.

One day he showed up at my house. When I saw him, I didn't know what to say or do. I thought to myself, "Mommy is here so nothing is going to happen." Then my mother told me that she was going to the store and would be back in half an hour. Jeff told my mother that he would stay and watch me for her.

"Do you want anything?" she asked me. I just told her to hurry back. When she left I got in my wheelchair. I thought if I stayed on the bed I wouldn't be able to stop him if he tried anything.

When I got in my chair he touched me on my leg. I pushed his hand away and told him, "You better stop. My mother is coming back soon." Then he went to touch my leg again. I didn't know what to do, so I froze up. Just as he was going to open my pants, we heard my mother talking to someone. He stopped and closed my pants up and told me not to say anything. Thank God my mother came in.

That Saturday I took my cousins Arnold and Elvin with me, so Jeff wouldn't be able to get me alone. He stopped going after me when he realized that I was always with my cousins. I started to hang up on him when he called me at home. I just got to the point where I couldn't take him trying to scare me any more, and I realized that he really couldn't hurt my family or me.

Careening Toward Kensho: Ruminations on Disability and Community

John R. Killacky

Waking up paralyzed from the neck down, I entered a new realm. Spirit, heart, and mind imploded as morphine, fear, and pain colluded. I tried to comprehend and name what had happened. Swelling and scarring from surgery to remove a tumor inside my spinal cord had miscircuited my body. Dawn was always the worst time, with the medical shifts changing; I was alone staring back at the world, fantasizing about getting to the window, breaking the glass, slitting my throat.

Two weeks postop, internal hemorrhaging thrust me back into intensive care. "Get Larry," I pleaded. I needed to see my husband. The burden was too much and I was ready to go on. Shortly thereafter he shook me back to consciousness and cried, "Don't die on me." I returned through his eyes, words, and breath. Blood transfusions stabilized me and a few days later I began the work of restructuring my body. One month later, Larry took me home in a wheelchair. Seven years later, we walk together careening from side to side assisted by a cane.

While still in the hospital, my husband spent each day loving me back to existence. He would read the headlines aloud, cheer on any slight progress in rehab, and play both hands of cards. Caressing my body that could not respond, often he would lie with me in bed, trying to soothe the blinding pain. One evening, he closed the curtains and kissed me. As he became visibly excited, I felt desirable again and hopeful that our life would return to a semblance of normalcy.

As someone who was quite phallocentric, I have been forced to reorient my sexuality. With almost no sensation in my genitals now, my only indication of an orgasm is violent spasticity in my left arm and

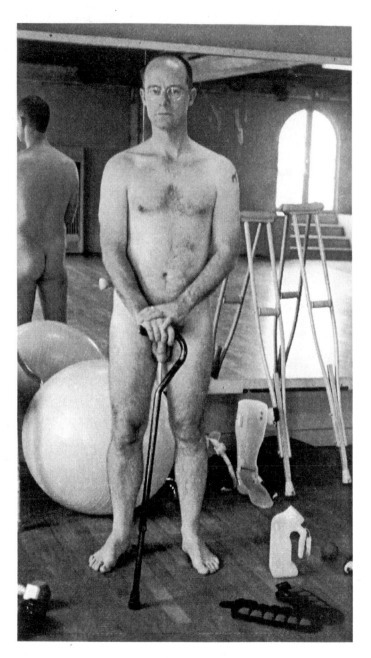

© 2001 by Laurie Toby Edison

leg. Reciprocating with my enfeebled fingers and locked-in neck is often very short lived. Yet the unconditional love of my husband has allowed new patterns to emerge; light massage and hugging are central to our relating.

Medical and therapeutic advice was nonexistent in this area—none of the hospital staff could tell us what kind of sexual function might return. Before discharging us, Larry and I spent an overnight in a transitional "apartment" on the medical floor, replete with videos designed for couples dealing with spinal injuries. The sexuality tape was beyond ludicrous. Not only was it completely heterosexual, it postulated that the ideal position for a man was still on top. It seemed more than a mere oxymoron for someone who has lost proprioception and feeling in the groin to be advised that thrusting and insertion still defined the sexual act.

As one way of connecting with other men coping with similar issues, I scanned the Internet and researched chat rooms and specialized newsletters for gay disabled men. Often I found the focus on the disability in many of these forums approaching a fetishistic level. In more than one personal ad, I was distressed to read "post-polio or missing limbs a plus." For many of the ads written by those differently abled, I found the self-loathing and desperate sense of isolation to be off-putting.

Determined to connect with other crips, I attended a disability arts conference to meet artists who had traveled from all over the United States and England. Blind and deaf people sat beside each other, worlds apart, waiting their turn to voice the injustice of existing within a hostile world. Actors railed against the inequity of being brought on location to teach "real" actors to mimic their actions. Artists who use wheelchairs wondered if they could play only their disability. As I joined others with stunted torsos, spastic limbs, and disconnected spinal cords, I was reassured that I was not merely my disability.

My questions nagged at random moments: *What to do with my anger? How to live with the ever-present pain? Will I ever stop wanting total recovery? How not to give up hope?* Everyone seemed so highly functioning and well-adjusted that I did not feel comfortable asking about despair and desperation. My husband Larry and I continue to grapple with ongoing depression. Before the surgery, we were very clear about acceptable alternatives. Even assisted suicide was discussed. Here, that topic was verboten.

I studied long-term survivors to see how their frames had adapted to changing circumstances, often by becoming increasingly bent. I was frightened to hear of overtaxed compensating muscles waning in exhaustion after decades of unrelenting service. Diminished mobility remains a daunting nightmare.

At this gathering, I was surprised to find internalized oppression subtly separating the *quads* from the *paras,* those with power chairs from those with manual chairs, even walkers from canes. Early-onset or congenital disabilities seemed more legitimate than degenerative conditions. We were divided by race, class, gender, and sexual orientation. One quadriplegic comic derisively parodied Siegfried and Roy for being so gay and the audience roared. My queer self was enraged at the homophobia and my walking self felt like a pretender as I left the conference.

As someone who has worked as an arts administrator for over thirty years, I found my profession no more accommodating of difference, especially regarding special needs. Despite the Americans with Disabilities Act legislation, I continually encounter inaccessible facilities and programs. Museums seem to be the most problematic. My gallery visits are now stamina based, not content driven. Are comfortable benches in galleries so contrary to the enjoyment of art? Group tours leave me behind; I often catch up just as the docent is leading the group on to the next room.

Recently when curating a visual arts exhibition, I was discussing its concept on the phone with one of the chosen artists whom I had not yet met. She insisted that her photographs were best seen when hung at her eye level. I reminded her of the ADA guidelines, and she retorted, "but those people don't come anyway." "Best practices might encourage more of us to attend galleries," I rebuked.

In alternative theater, music, and dance venues, I dread walking up and down rickety stairs. Once inside, I am angry at steeply raked seating with no railings and the only available handicap seating way off in the back or on the side. Mainstream theaters only place me farther from the stage. Afterward, I play a game of daredevil chicken with departing audience members as they impatiently bump and prod me. More than once I have been knocked over during an exodus.

Signed performances and assisted listening devices are now commonplace in theaters, yet it is still a radical notion to have audio description available for all the art forms. Visual artists, choreographers, playwrights, and composers are opposed to this kind of interpretation, fearing it would take something away from their work. However, these very same artists and their organizations have been unsuccessfully grappling with how to reach new and broader audiences.

Many colleagues try to be helpful, sometimes too helpful. Frequently, when I walk into a room, doors open, chairs move, and crowds disperse to make way for me. All this without me asking for help, which I have learned to do whenever necessary. Others refer to me in the third person; some assume I am mentally compromised as well. I bristled at one woman who runs an African-American museum as she told me that I must be grateful to my employer for taking a chance on me in my current state. Ignorance, fear, and prejudice take many forms.

Spirituality has been important during this time. I began sitting zazen with the late Zen master Isshû Miura Roshi in the late 1970s and have subsequently studied with various teachers, including the Tibetan leader, the Sixteenth Gyalwa Karmapa, Rangjung Rigpe Dorje. Decades of study and practice did prepare me, not always in expected ways.

Premorbid, Larry and I detailed our living wills. I did not want artificial life support. Believing that death was not an end, merely a transition, was enormously helpful. My single reluctance was attached to Larry: I still would not know how to ask his forgiveness if I was to go first.

Postmorbid, I found pain and frustration obscuring any sense of resolution and acceptance in meditation. Along the path of recovery, I often conjured Tibetan icon Mañjushri's sword, seeking to bring clarity to my confusion. I also reflected on the karmic implications of my paralysis, reconsidering my actions so as not to carry them forward.

While taking my first new steps, I was encouraged by Zen monk Thich Nhat Hanh's teachings about silent walking meditation, as well as Tibetan nun Pema Chödrön's reminders of always beginning from where we are right now. Simply placing one foot consciously in front of the other makes me more mindful of intention and consequence.

The holiness of my breath is underscored and impermanence illuminated, as I exist with the duality of body and spirit.

My relationship to the teachings has deepened, though I have lost my place in the community with which I sought refuge. Few temples and zendos are accessible, making it next to impossible for those of us who use chairs, walkers, canes, braces, or working dogs to join fully in prayer and contemplation. Not only would ramps, elevators, and chairs facilitate us meditating together, more thoughtfully conceived kitchens and gardens would allow us to work together.

Twenty years ago, my first teacher Isshû Miura Roshi spoke about *kensho* as "seeing into one's real nature through self-awakening in the body." Disability has given me opportunities to understand some of his wisdom. My connectivity to the world is deepening as I experience dependence on others.

Today as I continue to seek community, I search for hope as well. But even gallant Christopher Reeve, who once spoke about walking, now describes his life with a "before" and an "after." What I wanted to be temporary must be accepted as permanent. There is no choice in the matter, but I still long for the life before as I reconstruct the life ahead.

Repetitions

Raymond Luczak

Tired of asking "What was that again?"
I turn silent in their smoky presence.
I sit in the bar and stare at those men.

I am alone on Saturday night. Again.
Drink is a bitter solace; I have no defense,
tired of "Well, what did you say, then?"

I watch them nod their heads and laugh when
others throw whispers to fuel the suspense.
I sit in the bar and stare at those men.

Strobe lights strike lasers on those men
chatting. I maintain a mask's pretense,
tired of asking "What was that again?"

Silence and I are old childhood friends;
I turn off my hearing aids. My intense
eyes roam the bar and stare at those men.

They do not acknowledge me at all when
they leave with someone else. Again.
I sit in the bar and stare at those men,
who've tired of asking "What was that again?"

How to Find Love with a Fetishist

Bob Guter Interviews Alan Sable

Bob Guter talks to psychotherapist Alan Sable about the difficult dynamic between men who desire disabled men and the objects of their desire.

BOB: I understand that your perspective is not that of someone who "owns" the disability fetish, but the viewpoint of a professional and unbiased observer. Before we began running the tape, you put the discussion in context by observing that we're a fetishistic society across the board, whether we're gazing at sculpted pecs as a sexual fetish or drinking a ridiculously expensive bottle of Italian mineral water as a kind of socioeconomic fetish. Can you talk a little about some of the sexual fetishes we may be more familiar with, to give us a point of reference from which to start our search?

ALAN: I think there are two great components to a fetish. The first is predominantly visual, which comes across in the various "looks" we are familiar with in the gay world. In my time as a gay man it started with the Clone Look—that was a prime fetish—and the associated Leather Look. Those were definite looks, or fetishes, if you will. They are still around, but the look of the moment happens to be the Muscle Look. Clustered around the dominant look of the moment are the many variations that appear and reappear, like the Young Waif, the Grungy Guy, the Attractive-Younger-Guy-Who . . .

BOB: As you describe these variations I'm beginning to wonder: what is a fetish and what is merely a look?

ALAN: Exactly. Can an ordinary look be a fetish? I have been using the word fetish with gay abandon to make a point, which is that the word itself has a connotation—itself highly fetishized—which I, and I suspect many of us, have trouble with. It's a judgmental word growing out of a clinical perspective, one that says it's unhealthy by definition. We're stuck with a pejorative term, and I think its built-in negativity is a reflection of what the clinical word actually describes. It suggests that you fail to involve yourself with the real human being, that you're only involved with an external, superficial, visual thing. This is the heart of the clinical meaning of the word. And yet I suspect the tendency—which society defines as "unhealthy"—is programmed into us biologically as males. The content, however, varies: muscles this decade, mustaches the last.

BOB: So the tendency to fetishize is preprogrammed, you maintain, whereas content is more culturally and historically induced?

ALAN: Yes. And this is where I want to bring in the second great component of a fetish—one that I think is very important to talk about with respect to disabled men—and that's the emotional component, the emotional fetish, if you will. People have a very strong image—and I use that word to bring in the visual connotation, they have an image emotionally—of what is going to be fulfilling for them, even solve their problems. That emotional sense is even more fetishized, I think, than the visual. Sometimes it's feeling that I need a Big Strong Cop; it can be needing the Wonderful Husband, if you're into the domestic scene; or the Perfect Lover, if you're a Romantic. Another version is the Daddy, or alternately, the Son. And I think yet another version involves the Abled and the Disabled. Often the fetish is something we ourselves don't have, whether it's big muscles or a certain kind of "masculine" look. The do-have/don't-have contrast can be translated into connotations of "top" and "bottom." And, just as we can treat muscles as a fetish, we can treat ability the same way: the Sports Hero, for instance, is a society-wide fetish. Think of how his sweaty shirt is prized—is, in fact, fetishized.

BOB: The sweaty shirt that some guys would love to imagine masturbating over.

ALAN: Exactly! Ability is a socially-approved fetish, with those having less of it tending to fetishize it in those who have more of it. So, when we look at the nondisabled who fetishize the disabled, we find it's counter to, or the converse of, a dynamic that is a given fact in our society.

Keep in mind also that for every fetish there's a corresponding complementary fetish, or cofetish. For every Bottom there's a Top. The Waif Kid needs somebody to come along and pull his life together, so the Dad steps in to take charge. But just as the Kid (who may be chronologically no kid) needs the Dad, the Dad figure needs the Kid. I find this aspect a positive one, for reasons which I will go on to discuss.

In this discussion, we're interested in how physical disability, whether visible or not, becomes an emotional icon, or symbol for the fetishist. I think it's primarily because it's a way to care for someone, a way to approach someone vulnerable. Which is also saying it's a way to see someone as approachable. Just as gay men are attracted to the "masculine," partly because it's seen as powerful and even, in fantasy, invulnerable, all of which is easily fetishized, all that invulnerability and power is not always approachable, and so we find the emotional counterfetish that involves someone we can care for, the man who needs our help.

The person in need can be the Cute Young Kid with obvious needs, or the Big Hunky Guy who needs a good Husband/Wife behind him to keep the shirts ironed and the checkbook balanced. For essentially those same reasons, I think, some nondisabled men are prompted to love someone disabled, because that person is perceived as someone to be cared for. So in these ways I do not see the disability fetish as intrinsically strange, because it is constituted similarly to the others. But it must be comparatively rare numerically, which would explain why I never ran into it in twenty years of professional or social life.

BOB: Its comparative rarity may be hard to assess. I do know that you now can find a fair amount of disability fetishism online.

ALAN: Perhaps more people are coming out with this fetish than before. I'm sure it exhibits "dark" sides, too. Undoubtedly some nondisabled men feel, "Oh, I'm not very good-looking, but this disabled guy will find me appealing simply because I'm abled." Again, this sort of calculation would not be unique to the disability fetish. Another problematic side would be the nondisabled's stereotype of the disabled person as The Saint—and wouldn't it be wonderful if we could all marry Saints! This Saint-with-a-Disability will be a caring person, someone who has suffered a lot, a wonderful person who has overcome his disability, who has climbed Mt. Everest in a wheelchair, so imagine what he's going to do for me emotionally!

BOB: And furthermore he's going to be appealingly innocent sexually because he's had no experience.

ALAN: Right. Absolutely! He'll find me really hot; he'll appreciate me. I'm also hypothesizing that the fetishist of the disabled may also tend to be what I call an Emotional Top, someone who likes to be in control of the emotional field between himself and another; and that the disabled person, to respond to that fetish, has to be in some ways a Bottom, has to be someone who is going to be responsive to the emotional needs of this "more masculine" or more powerful person, the Abled person.

And so when you get a disabled person who does not have that personality, who doesn't have that interest, he's not going to respond to being fetishisized that way. Suppose he isn't a Saint. Or suppose he's the Emotional Top. He's not going to want to be fetishized in that manner—at any rate according to this hypothesis.

A further problem is that many disabled people are, in my experience, highly able, emotionally and physically. They can, in fact, take care of themselves very well, which does not make them good candidates for caretaking. Remember, fetishes have to fit. If you want to be a Cop and you want me to be a Robber, I have to find it in me to want to be a Robber. My guess is that the able-bodied man who fetishizes the disabled man is going to want to care for that person. But suppose the caregiver's emotional needs are too— shall we call it—top-heavy; the would-be caregiver may wrest security and power from the other's disability. He may want to give a lot but also control a lot. Turn up the darkness and dysfunction, and in that way the Helper can easily turn into a Nurse Ratched.

BOB: I had one very bad experience with someone who matched precisely the profile you're describing. It was hellish and it took me eighteen months to extricate myself from the relationship. He was exactly the controlling kind of Emotional Top you described, and I was not prepared to be the Emotional Bottom in the almost caricatured way that would have made him happy. And again, like you, I'm not talking about sexual mechanics at all, but much more subtle issues. He was determined to help me whether I needed it or not!

There's one incident I'll never forget. We were at a restaurant with two friends. In the past I had said to Danny, "You know, I really don't need any help cutting my meat" (even though I don't have much of a right hand). Well, it seemed I finally got this across to him. So there we four were and I ordered a whole lobster, which can be messy to handle even for people with the full complement of fingers. Noticing that I was having some trouble, the friend to my right asked, very casually, very appropriately, "Can I help with that?" To which Dan replied, loudly, too loudly for a public place: "You touch that lobster and I'll break your hand!"

ALAN: *He* wanted to do the lobster.

BOB: Or an even finer nuance: if he was prevented from helping me, nobody else was going to get away with it.

ALAN: That's a fine example of the absence of the complementary fetish: he obviously felt a need to take care of you in a way that you did not need.

BOB: In a way that I found demeaning. Alan, the way you're describing the disability fetish—as involving an Emotional Top with a need to take care of someone he sees as vulnerable—that seems terribly unappealing to me, since the whole dynamic is informed by a belief system that implies Disabled equals needing care. That equation is a real red flag for me.

ALAN: Yes. Like many disabled people you tend to be extremely able; you can indeed cut your meat. You've had, I imagine, to learn very consciously to do certain things that the rest of us take for granted. You're responsible; you like to do things for yourself, and you, like the rest of us, like to be in control.

So Danny was coming into direct conflict with your own need for power and agency. I imagine that kind of clash occurs frequently. That being said, I believe that most disabled men, like most people, want to be loved. And, like most gay men, I believe they want to be loved through their bodies. Now, while physical perfection seems a quintessential gay male icon—don't we, all of us, want to have powerful, sexy, perfect bodies . . . ?

BOB: Perfect, symmetrical bodies; I also think that the ideal of symmetry equaling beauty is something that's built into us.

ALAN: Yes, maybe biologically, as some think, and without a doubt culturally. That's an age-old image of beauty, at least in the West. If the disabled are not seen as symmetrical, they may not be seen as graceful, as powerful, as "perfect," and thus, by extension, as masculine. In the gay subculture, which fetishizes masculine beauty and perfection, disabled gay men have a problem from the start.

Now the "secret" that all therapists know is that all gay men, no matter how gorgeous, have been rejected many, many times, and are deeply wounded by that. Virtually all gay kids were rejected, even self-rejected, simply because of their gayness. And even if they grow up to be beautiful swans they still conceal an ugly duckling, the rejected part, which, in one way and another, continues to suffer rejection! Those gym-toned hunks are rejecting one another all the time. And, sometimes, we lesser mortals reject them.

BOB: We experience rejection not only in romantic love but rejection by parents, by straight peers, by other gay men, . . . by God.

ALAN: Then on top of all that, disabled gay men have various body types that are not now, never have been, and may well never be, seen as perfect, almost by definition. So given this perfection obsession that is so much a part of masculine fantasy life, disabled men are going to endure a double dose of rejection. Now here is where the big question, the startling question, arises: Is it possible that the fetish element might be useful to disabled men?

BOB: The answer you imply is: Yes, the disability fetish can be useful to us.

ALAN: It is a very radical-seeming idea. Let me try to lay out the basis of my inquiry. First, some qualifications: I am aware we haven't yet fully dealt with the problem of the disability fetish's inbuilt potential to lead to a clash over caregiving of the kind you experienced with Danny. I'm proposing we put that problem aside for a moment, to be looked at again later. The other qualification, of course, is that I'm aware that not all disabled men will be interested in nondisabled men. This inquiry will only be of interest to those who are.

But let us also remember that fetishes are important to gay men across the board. In fact, our whole culture is highly fetishized. In a funny way, disabled men have a built-in fetish for those who are into their disability.

BOB: The only problem being that a lot of us crips, maybe most of us, tend to be turned off by this fact. I've spoken to many guys who have found the attention of their nondisabled admirers a little bit, how shall I say this, "single-minded." Oh, hell, kinky is what I mean. One friend calls them the droolers. Another friend, an amputee, put it this way: "Love me, love my stump—but love me first!" His point being that he wanted to be loved for the totality of himself and that if his stump provided a jolt of additional sexual energy, great, but he does not want to play "also-ran" to his own stump.

ALAN: You know, and this is the point I would like us to consider: It may simply be a question of waiting for the shift in attention. In gay life, whether it's biceps or a mustache or glasses or crutches or a stump, I believe that the physical attraction—anatomical or prosthetic—nearly always comes first. Then, if it's longer than a one-night stand, the physically appealing parts begin to get folded into the whole personality, not the other way around. Of course, it can happen the other way around—the way I don't doubt many disabled men would prefer—but I strongly believe this is how it usually is for us gay men.

Don't we all look at the "fetish" first, then the person? One conclusion you could come to is: If someone is interested in what you've got, play that card. So my hope, my wish, for the disabled man is that he may achieve some measure of comfort in playing the card he has.

BOB: This *is* radical. If I understand you, what you're saying to disabled readers is: The disability fetish may be the road leading to the intimate relationship you want, so wouldn't it be useful if you could accept this kind of attention? Even more radical: from what you said earlier about corresponding cofetishes (the Daddy's Son, the Robber's Cop), are you wondering about men with disabilities actually getting into the fetish?

ALAN: Yes, it's all very well to be sitting here theorizing, but we are now down to the wire. This is where the disability fetish is different from the other fetishes. Let's look at that. Say you happen to have a big dick. You can certainly use that as your calling card. It's easy for you to use because you probably value a big dick, too. You think, "Ah, well that's sexy, and I've got one of those sexy things, so I'll use it." But if you're disabled, you probably don't think your "other stump," if that's your disability, is as sexy as that first one. You are probably not going to see it as a sexual thing, but as an object very, very different.

BOB: Speaking from experience, I can tell you you are absolutely right.

ALAN: So maybe it—whatever body part or "condition" the disabled owner is unhappy with—becomes in his own eyes unsexual, a reason for rejection.

BOB: Yes. Those body parts become emblems of shame and disgrace, never badges of erotic power.

ALAN: Exactly. Except to people—we've agreed for this conversation to call them fetishists—who are turned on by the stump or whatever other . . .

BOB: I think we've gotten hung up on stumps! Probably my fault . . .

ALAN: We've been using "stump" to stand in for the whole range of disabilities. It's a handy symbol because it's so phallic. The point we don't want to lose here is that the man who is turned on by certain physical parts or features has already sexualized them, whereas the chance that the disabled owner of those parts is going to eroticize them is small. To him they have a different meaning, probably a very antisexual meaning. They have been incorporated into the feeling that, "Gee, I'm not attractive, I'll never find someone." It's the part of his body that feels least erotic, even though to the admirer it may feel most sexual.

　　It's asking the disabled man to do a lot to eroticize, to fetishize, something he has antifetishized. Whereas if you're turned on by sculpted abs, it won't be difficult to find someone with those abs who thinks they're as sexy as you do, who wants to show them off, who wants you to admire them. As with the conflict over emotional dependence we talked about earlier, what we're describing is another way of talking about the lack of congruity between the admirer and the object of the admiration.

BOB: Those simple words sound painlessly clinical, yet what they describe is very, very painful to feel.

ALAN: Yes. And because this is so painful, and so crucial and specific, let me see if I can summarize where we are in this exploration. I believe that gay men often meet through a fetish. You like big cocks. I've got a big cock, we can make music. And then maybe we'll fall in love. So I do think that most gay men love the "cock" first and then the person. And that's easy to fetishize both ways, because everything in gay culture says "big-cock-equals-sexy."

But suppose I see you on crutches and a man with crutches is my ideal, for whatever reason in my personal history. But you think your crutches and perhaps your thin legs are ugly, so you won't be in a position even to try to understand my attraction. You may be frightened by my attraction. Your whole psychosexual history will be threatened by my interest because you have spent your life disidentifying with those parts instead of identifying with them. You and I may be disposed to like each other in a number of ways, but how on earth do we make music when we're in such emotional conflict on this pivotal issue? Is there even a way of getting through the issue?

BOB: I agree that this is the core question. It becomes less important, in practice, to ask where the disability fetish came from. It's more important to ask what we do about it and with it in terms of relationships.

ALAN: So, how do we continue the investigation? Where can we find the data? One of the things I would like to know—and I've never met people like this, but I believe we need to meet them and talk to them—is, what about disabled and nondisabled guys who make it, because their fetishes are complementary? The nondisabled guy who likes what the disabled guy has got and the disabled guy who likes his own stuff well enough so that he can say, "Yeah, let's go for it!"

BOB: I don't know how typical I am, but I've had experiences that cover some of this territory. With most of the men I've had sex with there was no reference, even implicit, to fascination (or revulsion) with my disabled status or particular body parts; however, I have made it with a small number of guys who flagged themselves as fetishists (though not one of them would have used that word, precisely because of the clinical, pejorative connotations you mentioned earlier). I met these guys through a personals ad many years ago, just after I had broken up with my partner of fifteen years.

Most of the men I met through that ad (which I ran in *Jarrod International,* a small, ahead-of-its-time personals publication, now defunct) I found incompatible. I found that they were, well, body-part obsessive is the only way I can describe it.

ALAN: You mean the disabled body parts?

BOB: Yes. Or missing body parts, or "disfigured" body parts. What I told myself at the time—and now I'm reexamining it all in light of this conversation—was that their particular interest didn't disgust me, it just didn't turn me on. More often than not, the single-mindedness of their approach bored me. Of course, a good part of it may also have been a kind of general incompatibility on other grounds, like music, food, and politics!

After about a half-dozen such misfires, I did connect successfully with someone who found me attractive for many reasons, including my disability. Raoul was a desirable partner for me for innumerable reasons; for one thing, he didn't focus on body parts or disability per se. Furthermore, he seemed not to obsess emotionally over those same issues in the way you and I were discussing earlier. We didn't have a conflict over caretaking. His concern that I didn't overtax my physical resources was something I came to accept as useful to me, and I didn't experience myself as on the bottom emotionally, perhaps because I knew how dependent he was on my caretaking in many, many areas of his life. By stumbling along together, by default and by practice, by talking to each other a lot, we found the kind of equilibrium that allowed us to function as a couple for quite a while.

ALAN: Maybe what your positive experience tells us is that the whole notion of fetish is oppressive, maybe we need to blur it out of existence. Perhaps we need to see that people have attractions we might at the present find unconventional, but the trick is to do what you and Raoul did, to allow time to subordinate those elements of attraction to the two people themselves, who are so much more complex and real. In that sense the feeling you mentioned earlier, "I come first and the fetish comes second" is valid. The fetish has to be subordinate to the relationship. But, as we have seen, it is also true, that the physical attraction, the fetish, usually comes before the relationship.

BOB: Sure. If I go into a bar, it's likely that the first man I find hot I'm attracted to because I like Roman noses and he's got the best example I've seen all week, not because I've chatted him up for half an hour first.

ALAN: Yes, exactly. Wherever on his body that "Roman nose" is! After all, the first thing we see is the first thing we see. In a situation like that, if you get from bar to bed you're still initially seeing him as an object. But even at that point the object is weighted with emotion. And certainly the objectified body of the disabled man is very weighted with emotion for both partners. But as we've noted before, it may be difficult to find congruent, complementary emotions that cluster around those desired objects, simply because most disabled men understandably prefer to have the fact of their disability, or its particular physical manifestation, noticed as little as possible.

BOB: Oh, yes! In fact some of us still try to pass whenever we can and however preposterous the success of that goal may be.

ALAN: And there's the conflict, the incongruity again. The disabled man is trying to hide what his would-be partner may find inherently desirable.

BOB: Yes, and, in my experience, it is not the only conflict attached to trying to hide my disability. I have noticed that I'm very much happier, more at ease when I'm over the stage of hiding, and here I'm not talking in the context of fetishists, but generally. When I was younger and in the market for sexual partners, I suffered great anxicty cruising somebody, but once we got past the point of shucking our clothes and getting into bed, for some reason I was OK.

ALAN: That's very interesting.

BOB: It's as if once we got past the preliminaries, I could feel enough confidence that the guy found something attractive about me, and then once I got rid of the wooden legs, with which I have a strong sense of being "not me" . . .

ALAN: Then it didn't matter.

BOB: Then it didn't matter, because what they're getting is really me and, at a certain level, difficult as it might be to reach that level, I'm comfortable with me.

ALAN: And I think that's really the key, Bob, your accessing your own level of comfort. As you remove parts, your prostheses, that are not really you, and present who you actually are, by that time you have enough confidence in yourself and your partner for the night, that you feel at ease, you can offer your Self, which is a great turn-on. But I think a lot of people disengage from what they're offering. Sometimes, for example, gay men almost literally become their cocks. Listen to the personals; a lot of them say: "I'm seven inches." They overidentify with the cock, they overfetishize it, and their partners do, too. So it becomes more like two body parts having sex instead of two people.

You know, underneath all this fetishistic disengagement from Self, I think one of our greatest difficulties, but one of our greatest desires, is to connect with another Self, something that doesn't come easily. When, having completed your undressing, you were suddenly offering your Self to that trick, that was very appealing, in fact, because ultimately he wanted that.

BOB: I can see that clearly now, although I don't think I saw it then, or at least not so clearly.

ALAN: I want to try again to go a little further here. I would like to suggest that, if you're comfortable with you, and if you are offering your Self, then it doesn't matter if the other person is fetishizing a part of you, because your Self permeates the part you're offering. I think it's possible to do both, to fetishize and to personalize, in parallel in the same relationship.

Now I have a question, or proposition to pose, which at this stage I will qualify as very tentative and simplistic. Maybe the key to success for disabled men who find themselves at the receiving end of the kind of attention we have been describing as the disability fetish is to offer the fetishized part, but to be sure to offer the Self with it. Admittedly, some fetishists will balk at that. They'll want only the part, because dealing with the human being is too complicated. This reminds me of what you said earlier about "droolers," those you see as absolutely unwilling or unable to connect. But I think even this can be reframed: I think almost every one of them would learn to connect, to personalize, if only given enough time. Of course, many will need much more time than most of their contacts would be able to stand, or would want to allow them.

BOB: You're saying: If guys with disabilities could only stand the drooling long enough, then . . .

ALAN: One day you might wake up and feel loved in a way that works. I humbly concede it's a very, very big *if,* presupposing an all-but-saintly capacity for bringing the Self, and the desire to understand the partner, to the relationship.

BOB: I think I understand what you're saying, and I believe that you're saying it not so much because you feel it's necessarily what we should do, but more to illustrate the map of the territory where, out of necessity, we disabled gay men find ourselves operating.

ALAN: Yes, exactly. It's less a should than a "what if?" There are many, many gaps remaining to be filled in. And the other thing I have of course been doing is focusing on the disabled man's side of the equation, principally because I have worked with a number of gay men with disabilities. We need to explore corresponding possibilities for behavior change on the part of the nondisabled fetishist. I'm sure of this, but, as I've said, I have never met such a person and, at this stage, can only speculate.

BOB: Many of the personals ads I've read seem to cry out for understanding, but one aspect puzzles and irritates me: why are so many of these men so stuck on fetishizing particular and only particular disabilities? "I'm not interested in quads, thank you very much, I'm interested only in CPs with black hair and mustaches who use crutches, *not* a wheelchair." Doesn't this make a mockery of the attempt to find someone? How many potential responders can possibly exist?

ALAN: It gets so narrow, right. But on the other hand, with the Internet and other more widely accessible sources of communication, there's a new sort of reality at work. You can find niches, sometimes. People do. The personals listings in your Web 'zine, *Bent,* might allow people the chance to find exactly what they desire, at least in terms of the category of person. And that can be just as true for your disabled advertisers as it is for the nondisabled ones. There's a big leap from the category to the actual person, but it's a start.

Given that caveat (and without minimizing its importance), I believe that something like the Internet is a much better vehicle than, say, the bars. My understanding is that cruising the bars is fraught with complications for gay men with disabilities.

BOB: Yes. If I, obviously disabled, walk into a bar and cruise somebody I think is hot, what if he returns the look? I don't know if he's interested in my cruise or merely curious about my appearance.

ALAN: Right. Obviously physically disabled people are used to attracting attention. It's confusing because bar etiquette says that if you're looking, you're interested, but you can't assume that. If he's looking, he might not be interested; and conversely, because the disabled in our society are stigmatized, an interested nondisabled man might be embarrassed to make an overture, for fear of being associated with the stigma. So, if he's not looking, he may yet be interested.

BOB: That's very true. Either way, many of us are sensitive to approaches from the nondisabled. We can be hard to cruise by them. Broadside targeting of disabled men by nondisabled men can be an instant turnoff. Too many unpleasant associations.

ALAN: He may or may not be a drooler . . .

BOB: But the disabled guy is all too likely going to assume, "Oh, no. Another idiot. Another pity monger. Another creep."

ALAN: Yes. I've been acquainted with enough disabled people in therapy to recognize that as a powerfully negative counterstereotype, arising for reasons which are very, very understandable: disabled people are subjected to all kinds of undesired approaches. And yet I think it's important for the guy in the chair to be prepared to relinquish that stereotype, because the particular nondisabled guy in question may or may not be a creep.

What is so striking to me about the disability fetish is that it's not the "normal" one; you're not supposed to have this one. This tells me that the person has something interesting about him, he has his own agenda that's specific, one that's not the usual prepackaged agenda sold to us. Now I think there's already evidence of sensitivity in that agenda, something of caring for a person, which is positive. And surely courage is something the fetishist must also have. He's taking a risk, as you point out, simply by approaching the object of his desire.

All of this tells me that there has to be a vulnerability to the person with this fetish, which we are inclined—for well-known reasons—to overlook. Even though we don't understand it at present, is it too much to ask disabled men to grant their admirers at least the acknowledgment of some underlying vulnerability?

BOB: You have come up with another radical concept. That we may be so busy nursing our own vulnerabilities that we don't see anyone else's. The concept of "I'm not the only vulnerable person around here" certainly would tend to make the playing field more level. And it appears to tie in to some degree with what I said earlier about the many ways in which, with Raoul, I was the one looking after him. His vulnerabilities were accessible to me.

ALAN: Yes. It seems it may feel easier when you can take onboard the possibility that the other guy has something he needs help with. Perhaps this is the hidden other side of the moon. So you might begin by trying to diminish your prejudice toward the fetishist, at least enough to test some of what I've been saying, by talking to these people, seeing what they're like.

BOB: By recognizing that they're not all creeps. But another challenge is the small number of men we're dealing with—a minority within a minority within a minority. Suppose a guy finds me attractive because I'm an amputee. So we go out for coffee and it turns out he's an opera queen and I'm a Forty-Niners fan, he likes red meat and I'm a vegetarian.

ALAN: Granted. Although to pursue my point, I think this is precisely where the most useful testing can take place, in conditions where thoughts of romance have been abandoned. One of the absolutely most difficult things we face as gay men is making friends when one of us rejects the other sexually. That becomes a very hard friendship issue. We can only do boyfriends, tricks, lovers, and girlfriends. It's hard for us to befriend someone who rejects us sexually.

BOB: Very hard.

ALAN: Yes, but it might be very useful—and interesting. Remember, it cuts both ways. It's equally hard for someone we reject. After all, what have you and I been talking about but a disabled man who rejects a fetishist? He may in fact be especially vulnerable to such rejection. Now, might it be valuable for that disabled man to say to his suitor, "Look, I'm not interested at all in going to bed with someone who fetishizes my disability, but I'd like to get to know you and find out what makes you tick."

Here is where the other side of the equation comes in: surely this is where the fetishist has to be willing to make his leap in the direction of confronting those things which make him most vulnerable. Surely if he's sensitive, intelligent, and a little bit experienced, he'll be interested in learning to stop the exaggerated behavior you've called drooling and look at the realities of forging a relationship. So we come to see that what I said earlier was too simplistic. We see now that, if it is our hope for the disabled man to gain greater comfort in his dealings with the fetishist, we must also expect the fetishist to try to become comfortable with exposing his vulnerability to scrutiny.

I think these questions are not just rhetorical or hypothetical. From what I know about disabled gay men it seems they tend to think their best prospects are with men who just don't care about the disability, it's just not an issue, because they have so much else in common—interests, personalities, styles—that a disability is a minor dimension. Their hope is to find these men in the course of ordinary social life, which may include some forays into gay bars. Now, this is an attractive goal. But the problem of the minority within a minority within a minority applies here too. And what do you do while you're waiting to find just that right niche?

BOB: Your analysis invites only one reply: Step out of the box you've put yourself in. Try your luck testing encounters with, among others, some of the people we've agreed to call fetishists.

ALAN: Not breaking through the impasse seems to me like settling for less. You see, and this is a kind of hobbyhorse of mine, I also want to say that I think the bars are rotten venues for disabled men. In fact, they're rotten venues for anybody who's looking for a relationship. Now one of the problems with what I've just said is that disabled men want sex, too, so why not go to a place where it's easy to find? But as a psychotherapist, I'm also saying (and this doesn't always go down well in the gay community) that love is more important than sex. And it's also true that disabled men are not going to do as well, in general, in the purely sexual arena.

As I see it, they need to say to themselves that that arena, the arena where guys are looking only for the stereotypical Body Beautiful, is not one where I may expect to excel. But who knows what I can do in the emotional arena? Now, this may seem ironic, but I think that disabled gay men's best chances in the emotional arena lie on the other side of the impasse presented by the disability fetish. This is because—and I wish I knew more about this so I could make a stronger case—but my guess is that the fetishizers of the disabled are going to be very strong and interesting people emotionally, as indicated by the fact that they haven't fallen for the standard fetishes.

They probably have a strong caring element, which is a valuable human capacity. They are persistent in the face of the rejection and the prejudice they encounter from disabled and nondisabled alike, which shows how very important and emotionally driven are their desires and their underlying vulnerabilities.

BOB: In my experience the caring sometimes doesn't show through the single-minded persistence.

ALAN: The potential negative character we mentioned earlier is the possible control-freak aspect, but lots of people have that anyway, without the disability fetish! What I'm saying is: disabled men are probably going to do better going for the gold, the solid, emotional connection with a partner, than they are going for the silver, the superficial attraction of sex with such horny men as may be culled from the bars. I think that we have, between us, made at least a case for the idea that a vein of solid, relational gold exists within every fetishist. As I see it, this gold offered by the fetishist may be more available to the disabled man than either the silver or the other gold, that harder-to-find lucky strike offered by men who are both congenial and have an entirely neutral stance in relation to disability.

BOB: And how do you answer those who respond by saying, "This is all so much psychobabble. These people with the disability fetish are *sick*!"

ALAN: I would say this is a legitimate and understandable point of view, but you should know I think it will keep you this side of the impasse we have described, and I would invite you to look at what the implications are for you of keeping yourself on this side. To the extent that you are on the lookout for sickness, you will fear it and see it, and find it, and label it, and it will be real. And you will be doing exactly what nondisabled society does to the disabled.

If your greater interest is to look for connection, you will find that this inevitably means becoming curious about taking on some other guy's emotional baggage, finding that it's connected in some way with your own, and both of you somehow learning to bear the joint burden.

Loving You Loving Me

Samuel Lurie

My lover asks for a copy of a photo of me that somehow didn't make it into the stack of doubles I sent in the mail. These are pictures I can barely stand to look at and I know that, to my partner, they capture many of the things he loves about me. But I instinctively turn away from pictures of myself, learned from a lifetime of seeing only ugliness in the mirror.

I was born and raised as a girl, but not a normal one. No one close seemed to really mind my tomboy ways, a tacit acceptance that was a stroke of luck. But still, I felt destined to be forever misunderstood, unable to ever name the reason for my sense of shame and wrongness. I developed a hefty armor to shield myself from tormentors, and I became pretty good at standing up for myself. But the shame of absolute difference ran into my bones, my pores, my essence. I couldn't name what it was, but I didn't need to. It was doing its damage without benefit of a common language. I got the message, lived the message, that my queer body, butch body, freak body, was barely entitled to take up any space at all.

Thankfully, I did do a lot of work to break out of that space, but it hasn't been along a straight, continuous line. Three years ago, I traveled to San Francisco for chest reconstruction surgery, and that was a big step in making my body right. But when I came back from surgery, I confessed to the friends who took me home from the airport, "now who's gonna want me?" I finally had the body I dreamed of, or part of it anyway, but couldn't quite imagine anyone else wanting it. As I settled into my body, a lot of things shifted and I could believe, if only for a second at a time, that I could be attractive. But I still wasn't sure to whom. I mean, what category could I possibly use to place my personals ad? How could I describe who I was, who I was looking for?

I want to add, though, that this wasn't done in isolation. There are many of us challenging the gender binary, creating a new language, new words for who we are and what we want.

Perhaps it is no surprise that I found a poet.

I met Eli at a reading and, for me, it was love at first paragraph. We kissed at lunch and spent that first night together. All faster than either of us had ever experienced and at the same time shockingly safe. I don't want to gush too romantic, though you can probably tell I could. To put it simply, we began to find a home in each other's bodies, in our intertwined bodies, in our own bodies being touched like this for the very first time.

Eli too had to move through layers of shame, embarrassment, complete unfamiliarity. He had never let his tremoring hand loose on someone else's body before, had always tried to hold it back. I guess I gave him more than permission. Immediately, my body started begging for that exact tremoring touch. When I discovered that his right hand tremored more than the left, that's the one I pulled to me, to rub my chest, cheek, thigh. I didn't want a single bounce to go to waste. I don't want to sound objectifying, or fetishistic, as if I was only attracted to this person because of the shake. But I think that there was an utter magic in the combination of my wanting that very specific thing that for Eli was the root of so much of his own struggles with his body. I wanted it, loved it. More than acceptance—it was an active desire.

Of course we can't easily explain desire—why it's there or where it comes from. But being desired, and trusting that, reciprocating that, cracks us open. Sensually, to me, Eli's CP is literally a gift. And I recognize the absurdity of trying to imagine: would I have fallen in love with Eli if he didn't have CP? That's an unanswerable koan. Would a boulder be a boulder if it wasn't a boulder? I fell in love with someone with CP, and I like the CP. Can it be that simple?

Eli once wrote: "Me, looking at me in the mirror and liking what I see, is a minor miracle." We have helped each other achieve this miracle, and it feels more than minor. In part that has come from the affirmation of the observing eye. But it has also crept up from within. Pride and self-love become mighty powerful by-products of being admired and loved. Someone has to do a lot of convincing for us to be able to peek at the mirror. And we still have to do a lot of work ourselves.

For instance, what work did Eli have to do to accept help from me? On one of our first hikes in Vermont, on a steep, slippery trail, the kind where Eli moves especially slowly—he was shrugging off my outstretched hand, not wanting any help. But I was only offering it in part to provide balance. "We're lovers out on a hike," I reasoned, "you're supposed to want to hold my hand." He laughed, relaxing, the tension breaking. Eli has spoken of the filters that work to keep it all out. Here was one mighty big filter doing its job.

We hike more easily now, Eli referring to my hand serving as that "third point of contact"—stabilizing and comforting. But he still gets self-conscious of his preference for crawling on all fours across narrow bridges, or dropping to his butt to slide down even short descents over rocks. A key to learning how to be okay with who we are is to have others not judge us. I have no investment in how he crosses a bridge or uses a foothold. Each hike, maybe, takes him a little further toward believing that. He's got nothing to prove to me.

My capacity to not judge frees him. And his capacity to not judge frees me. So, let me tell you how my crip/queer/tranny lover helps me overcome my shame. I spoke earlier of my queer, tranny, freak self. A lifetime with psychic armor as sure as skin. Rooted with shame, with a notion that this butch, tranny, freak body could never be desirable or hot. A shame that is embedded in the collective unconscious of gender-nonconforming queers, where thousands of daily encounters are layered with danger, disgust, or distress.

Having transitioned, I am hardly done. Yes, I am more at home in my body. Yes, I am safer on the street, more solid in everyday relationships. Less visibly challenging the gender binary, and less likely to have to pay a price for that publicly. But the shame I speak of cannot possibly go away in real time. It feels as if it precedes my very being, going back into a psychic prehistory. A lifetime where I could never settle in to anything normal, couldn't pursue a "normal" job, have "normal" relationships. Any attempts I made fell so far short they seemed like mockery. What my body looked like, what my body wanted, could not be easily explained. I had to stay small. Somehow, a big part of unlearning that need to stay small has come from my relationship with a person who not only loves every single part of me, but who is also committed to moving at an intentionally slow pace, perhaps immeasurable in human time. I have always survived by moving with a kind of mania, a rushing around that, ironically (maybe), has kept me from freaking out. But it's the slowing down that I really needed.

On that same early hike where Eli first took my hand, he gazed around at the Vermont ruggedness, cliffsides of granite, quartz, and shale. Giant rocks dotting the hills, dropped long ago by glaciers moving through. "If I believed in reincarnation," he said, "and I had a choice? . . . I'd want to come back as a boulder." And there we had it. To me, Eli is a boulder, a bedrock, a stabilizing force that took a long time to get there and isn't going anywhere fast. What does his CP have to do with this utter stillness? How does his perpetually tremoring body also define an essence of solidness, of nonmovement? Perhaps this is just one more example of how contradictions create completeness.

Here are a few of my contradictions: I am a man who was born female. As a gay transman, I am a faggot without a dick. And no matter what they say about normal, about possible, here I am. I know *I exist.* How do we create a language to normalize who we are? Just how do we take hold of our unique bodies, reframe a lifetime of shame into one of comfort and pride? How do we actively love and celebrate, not just accept, our unique selves?

I do not pretend to be able to answer these questions.

Yeah, it helps when we have a lover who says we're fucking hot. Or have a good exchange at a bar or on the street. But it's a tenuous little bead of confidence that can disappear in the moment it takes someone to turn away from a wink.

But I know that when I look at pictures of my boyfriend, the ones he winces at out of lifelong habit, I stare transfixed and hungry. And now he knows that too when he smiles toward the camera lens. And for myself, I want to be as beautiful as my lover thinks I am and I grow taller by being loved by him. As old and as thick as a glacier, this pain is rooted deep. Every kiss and shaky caress are like years of sun beating down to begin to melt away layers. I know we do this for each other. A desire that has no qualifiers, no "in-spite-of," or "although." We are discerning, critical people and we want each other for all the things that we are. Crip, tranny, queer. No judgments. Just love. Freaky, wonderful, real love.

In so many ways, I am truly grateful.

A Meeting with George Dureau

Max E. Verga

> The photographer and his subjects have entered into a shared
> enterprise, whose purpose is to record not only outward appear-
> ances, but an inner sense of worth in the person being photo-
> graphed—achieved sometimes against overwhelming odds.
>
> Edward Lucie-Smith on George Dureau

Several years ago, photographs by George Dureau accompanied
an article I wrote for *Drummer,* a magazine designed for fetish and
S&M enthusiasts. As a regular *Drummer* contributor, I had always
tried to stretch boundaries by including characters that did not fit the
usual overendowed stud image. Titled "Different Bodies," my article
explored the relationships between able-bodied men and men with
disabilities. *Drummer* built a feature, "Maimed Beauty," around the
story and then decided to add photographs by George Dureau.

The magazine received more letters about "Maimed Beauty" than
any other feature. Partly in response to those overwhelmingly positive letters, I wrote another piece about disability, this time fiction,
called "Chester." *Drummer* published that, too, also with illustrations
by George Dureau.

George is a New Orleans artist who often photographs local men
with disabilities. Since I'd already decided to visit New Orleans, I
thought I'd track him down and try to arrange a meeting. True to the
tradition of Southern hospitality, I found myself invited to his home
for lunch. George lives in the lower part of the French Quarter in an
area once notorious for drug deals in the park facing his house. By the
time I got to see it, the neighborhood had reverted to its earlier, quiet
state. I even saw a few yuppies in the park.

I had expected that I might be met by one of George's models, but
the man who ushered me inside, George's strikingly handsome assistant, had no observable disability. As I walked upstairs I noticed some

works in progress on the walls, stylized portraits of dwarfs that would later be the basis for a book of George's paintings. The rooms had an open feel, obviously arranged to accommodate his work. When I reached the second floor I recognized George immediately from the photo of him and his frequent subject B. J. that had been included in "Different Bodies."

George is African American and his tastes run toward other African-American men, especially those with disabilities. The majority of men he photographed for his first book are locals, many from the poor neighborhoods circling the Crescent City. Other subjects included a number of dwarf wrestlers and a few men from other cities. Our conversation touched on the lives of his models, including the legless B. J., whose arms-akimbo pose in *Drummer* had sparked questions about his body. There were those who wondered if he possessed sex organs or normal bowel functions. George showed me a photo of B. J. with an American flag draped tightly across his loins. The photo left no question about B. J.'s sex organs.

B. J., George explained, had been born with flippers emerging from drastically shortened calves. For "aesthetic" reasons, the flippers had been surgically removed, leaving extensive scarring. B. J. used a skateboard for mobility. It did not seem that George and B. J. had been involved in any way other than model-artist. It did not even seem that B. J. was gay or bisexual.

The photographs of B. J. were representative of George's work, ragged-edged, black-and-white portraits lacking background detail, which forces the viewer to focus attention on the subject, often portrayed naked. George presents disability without visual comment or apology. Only one other time would I see such powerful depictions of disabled men, at a Seattle exhibit that featured medical photographs of Civil War veterans taken to document the effects of war.

George told me of searching for models in hospital wards, on Bourbon Street, and in parts of the city that most tourists never see. I've seen some of those areas and I understand their sadness: They will always yield men with disabilities by reason of the poverty and neglect found there.

It was hard not to be impressed by the beauty of George's photos and the desirability of his subjects. One of the amputees George photographed had been his lover. Another man, also a former lover, was someone I encountered years after my meeting with George. Yet another is a famous little man who frequently can be seen at Mardi Gras time in full leather, accompanied by his multiply pierced lover.

Beautiful as they were, the photographs only hinted at the sexual power of the men they depicted, something I learned years later, after making love to several of the same men. Unlike the photographs of Diane Arbus, which emphasize the grotesque qualities of her subjects and their uneasy relationship to society, George Dureau's photographs suggest nobility.

In one, an African-American man uses a stick to maintain his balance while crossing his stump over his undamaged leg. The viewer is forced to acknowledge the discrepancy between the two limbs, but that discrepancy is merely part of a portrait that includes a wild mane of hair, the fineness of the subject's torso, and the impressiveness of his exposed sex. The viewer is forced to look at the obvious pluses and what some would call minuses and come away weighing both as reasons for either rejecting or embracing the image.

The same holds true for George's image of Wally Sherwood. Wally is a man with a strong, beautiful face; his arms and legs defy ordinary proportions and thus say "dwarf." But if you equate "dwarf" with "undesirable," that beautiful face (and a well-packed jockstrap) may convince you to reevaluate your preconceptions. Wally is a sexual being, one not above standing naked on a bar as one man after another confirms just how desirable he can be.

The fact that many disabled men have exposed themselves to George's camera may be a tribute to their courage. But the fact that George Dureau has photographed them in a way that makes his belief in their beauty unmistakable challenges us to think hard about the kinds of beauty we are used to extolling.

George and I talked for hours and he showed me photographs that had not made it into his book. There was a little man from Atlanta, a very hot-looking lawyer, whose friends insisted he pose for George. And so he did. I had seen him once during a visit to Atlanta and was impressed by his handsomeness. There were photos of another little man with patrician looks and seemingly mismatched limbs. A bare-chested man with a prosthetic arm hook draped across his chest was someone I had seen coming out of a gay bar in Chicago.

Sadly, George's books are hard to come by these days. A trip to a local gay bookstore will net dozens of albums of well-muscled men in exotic surroundings, often engaged in equally exotic acts. Few of those models reflect the people who buy the books and even fewer offer bodies that challenge our perceptions about what is perfect and what is desirable.

I don't know if George Dureau's mission to photograph those other bodies grows out of his own sexuality or the need to shock. Most likely his motives combine the two. I met George only once. Since then I have seen one or two of his photographs on Web sites that featured pictures of disabled men. Some people protested that such photos objectified men with disabilities in a negative way. Most sites have stopped using them, mostly because of copyright issues. To me, it seemed incredibly positive that for a short while pictures of disabled men were given equal play on the Internet alongside pictures of hunks and bodybuilders.

Perhaps if more of George's photos had made it onto Web sites, disabled men themselves would have been able to view the images in a new way, as something that gives pause, stimulates in unexpected ways, and manages to put men with different bodies, clothed or unclothed, on an equal footing with the stereotypical "normals."

Face Value:
Text for a Performance Piece

Karl Michalak

It all started
when I went into that big high-priced hospital
in the busy City of Death.

Something was wrong with my face,
or at least that is what everybody told me.

You see, I came from a place
in the hinterlands up North
and at that time
there were no doctors there
who knew how to handle my particular condition.

I have no way of knowing exactly how the trouble started.
I do know my mother had a difficult pregnancy
and that they gave her all kinds of drugs
to force her to carry to term.

They gave her all kinds of drugs
with very strange names.
To keep her from losing the baby
that her body didn't seem to want.

This was in 1958.

"Face Value" has been edited from a longer version that Karl never got to perform.

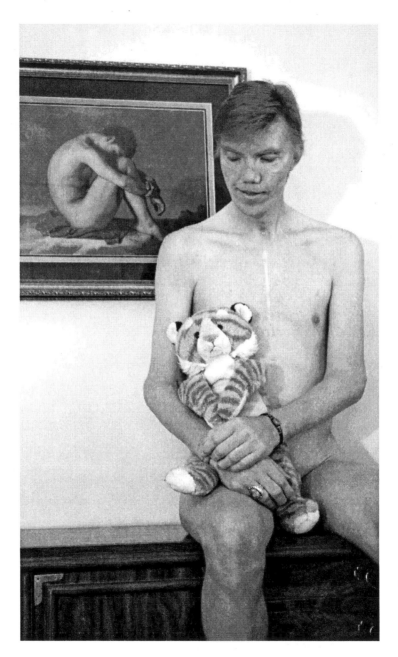

© 2001 by Laurie Toby Edison

The doctors seemed to belong
to the "all life is sacred/save the fetus at all costs" school.
They did this because
to do anything else would have been a sin.

The doctors did all this
until my mother developed toxemia,
which caused her to swell up
and practically killed her.

They did all this, they said,
because being a mother
was her function as a woman.
Or at least that is the story
that they told her.

And then of course there was Red Skelton.
One day when I was about two
I saw something funny on *The Red Skelton Show.*
I don't remember exactly what it was.
I only remember that I laughed so hard I
fell backwards in my chair.
The seat of the chair hit me in the face
and that was the end of me.

At the emergency room
my father refused to spend money on X-rays.
The doctors who supposedly knew everything
said everything was OK.

This was the first of many lies
that the doctors were to tell me.

I found out later
when I was much older
after all the damage had been done
that I had suffered a lateral fracture of my upper jaw.

This led to other complications
all because nobody bothered to take an X-ray.

Or perhaps because my father, who worked in a GE plant,
couldn't or wouldn't spend the extra money.
Everything healed up
but in a very strange way.
Years later
when it was very obvious
that something was very wrong with my face
everyone
said one or more of the following:

It's the Lord's will.
Just learn to live with it.
It's all in your imagination.
Don't be so self-centered.
Shut up and do your homework.
Other people are worse off than you.

So many years later
after I begged them to do something—
anything—
I was sent to the high-priced hospital
in the busy City of Death
many miles away
to figure out where they had gone wrong.

The doctors in the high-priced hospital
in the busy City of Death
said that they could help me
but that because I had no money,
that is, not enough to be a private patient
I had to go through a clinic
frequented by the poor.
And when I got there
something went very wrong, you see
and now here I am
telling you this story.

Because I had no money
I had to do it their way.
I had to beg to be helped.
I had to insist on it.

And as I was to learn over and over again,
after the damage was already done,
nothing flies in this fucking world
unless you have money
or until you get angry.

And there's one more thing:
Everyone tells me that I asked for it.

Leave well enough alone, they said.
You don't look so bad.
But I knew better.
I knew it wasn't all in my imagination.
I knew every time I looked in the mirror
that something was very wrong.
But because I was a child
nobody would believe me.

It took me many years
to get the help that I needed
and then
after I was butchered by the doctors
in that very busy hospital
in that very expensive City of Death
it took me many more years
to fix it again.

I know what some of you are thinking.
You think I'm just dramatizing
or exaggerating for effect
or crying in my beer
or feeling sorry for myself.

All right.

Maybe my imagery is exaggerated.
But I don't think so.
Not by much.

I remember very clearly
what it was like in surgery
there in that busy hospital
in the City of Death.

They had shaved my head the night before
the way they do in prison movies
about condemned murderers
headed for the electric chair.

Before they knocked me out
I remember how cold it was.
It was so cold that it made me want to pee.
There were bright lights
and classical music
playing from somewhere.

(You see, the doctor who butchered me
 had very sophisticated tastes.)

And rows and rows of surgical instruments.
Scissors and pliers and all kinds of things.
And something called a Stryker Saw
which I later learned is used
for cutting up corpses in medical schools.

Later on
I read somewhere
that when Joseph Mengele
sent people to the gas chambers in Auschwitz
there was always somebody
playing classical music
in the background
just like in the movies.
Just like in those surgical suites
in the very busy hospital
in the busy City of Death.

I laughed when I heard that.
I don't know why.

I couldn't see because my eyes were swollen shut.
I couldn't hear out of one ear because it was full of blood.
I couldn't walk because without any prior consent of mine
they had taken some bone out of my hips
and used it to put my face back together.

So they doped me up
and cleaned me up
and sat me up in intensive care
with a lot of pillows.

I didn't feel any pain.
Because my head was swollen up
to such outrageous proportions.
It was like something on
Outer Limits,
Fright Theatre,
or one of those horror movies
I used to watch.
Edema, they called it.

My mother came in.
I knew she was there
even though I couldn't see her.
For a long time she was very quiet.
I remember that because I couldn't talk
I had to spell things in her hand.

Two minutes later
I started hemorrhaging all over the place.

After it was all over
we wanted to sue the doctors
but by that time they had dispersed or disappeared
to other parts of the country
to work in other very expensive hospitals
in other very busy Cities of Death.

The lawyers in my hometown
up North in the hinterlands

said that I probably did have a case.
But they wanted five hundred dollars
for retainer fees, they said,
before they could initiate proceedings.

My father didn't have five hundred dollars.
Or at least, if he did, he wouldn't spend it.
Instead of spending money
he went down to the cellar
and turned on the ham radio
and started talking to strangers
about the weather in Wisconsin.

Somewhere around this time
I quit going to church.
Everyone in the church told me:
We are meant to suffer in this life.
It's God's will.
Just learn to live with it.
Surely I was being punished for some great sin.

But I figured
any god who would allow a thing like this
to happen to me
can't be worth too fucking much.

And I still think so.

Because every time I read the newspaper
every time I watch the news on TV
I hear a story about somebody else.
Somebody else
who went into that high-priced hospital
in the busy City of Death
and never came out again.

And I realize I am lucky
to have gotten away with my life,
even as mangled and misfired as it is.

To take my mind off all of this surgery
I went to the movies.
And on the movie screen I saw
all kinds of people:
crippled people,
deformed people,
paralyzed women with pretty faces,
drug addicts,
homosexuals,
criminals,
and women who were raped.

They were all lumped together
in one huge category
called Undesirable.

Years later I went to a major university
in the high-priced City of Death
to find out how these movies were made.

Five years and twenty-five thousand dollars later
I still don't understand anything.

Every once in a while
somebody gets an Oscar
for playing one of these undesirable people
and everything seems to be all right again.
Look, look, the undesirable ones say,
everything is getting better.
They're paying attention to us.
But not for long.

Because up there at that high-priced hospital
in the busy City of Death
business goes on as usual.

I'm not the only one, you see.
I'm not the only one.

I know this because
while I was stuck at home recovering,
while I was traveling around the world,
while I was hanging around in bars
in the City of Death
learning all too well how to drown my sorrows
I began to hear stories.

There was the young girl
who went to the emergency room
of that big high-priced hospital
in the City of Death.

She had a series of known allergies
but nobody in that emergency room
bothered to look at her chart
so she was given drugs
in strange combinations
which caused her to have seizures
and die.

And then there was the famous artist,
the one who made art out of soup cans.
Everyone loved the pictures he made
of ordinary household objects
and beautiful celebrities.

He went into that big high-priced hospital
in the busy City of Death
for routine gall bladder surgery
and never came out again.

Finally there was the man
who liked to make puppets
and made millions of dollars.
Everyone thought he was wonderful
because he made people laugh.

They said he had pneumonia
and when he died

they said it was all his fault
because he should have come in earlier.

This is an increasingly familiar tune.

They blamed it on the nurses,
all of whom were women,
or they blamed it on the patients,
all of whom were powerless.

They blamed it on everyone but the doctors.

And in the meantime
at that very high-priced hospital
in the busy City of Death
business goes on as usual.

And now everyone asks me
Why are you doing this to yourself?
Why are you rubbing your nose in it?

Because I know now that
I am not exceptional.

I know now that my situation
is not unusual.

Because I'm not the only one, you see.
I'm not the only one.

I have no identity now
as anything other than a disease carrier.
The language which other people use
to describe my predicament
has been simplified over time
so that now I am no longer "HIV positive."
I simply "am HIV."
As if there were no distinction at all
between the disease and myself.

We are one and the same,
inseparable.

Someday I'm gonna make my own goddamn movie.
It'll be a Technicolor extravaganza
full of faggots and lesbians and whores
and drug users and blacks and Hispanics
and AIDS patients and HIV positives and homeless people.

The discarded of the universe
who comprise every level of society's junk heap.

They'll glitter up there on the silver screen
wearing their rejection like a badge of honor
and in the final reel
they'll turn their guns on Washington
and the doctors
and the lawyers
and all the other bullshit shovelers
whose laziness and money grubbing
have perpetuated this disaster.

The complacent, flawless, perfect ones
will go down in a hail of gunfire
and all those who have been abused and thrown away
will rise up as one
and live happily ever after
if only for one more minute.

Amen.

Acting for Others, Acting for Myself

Michael Perreault

I'm a child of the 1960s. I saw plenty of antiwar and civil rights stuff. I took part in some demonstrations, but I was never an activist. I saw people beaten up; I saw a man's face ground into the pavement with a burning cigarette still in his mouth. I decided that that was not my way of doing things, but I felt guilty about it. I felt I should be doing more, paying back to society. And I realized that that feeling was coming from my own place of inadequacy.

Then, in the 1970s, the consciousness-raising group I participated in taught me that simply being an out gay man, a man who made love to another man, was a revolutionary act in itself. That's when I realized, too, that only actions I take on my own behalf can be the seeds of a larger activism, whatever form that might take.

The conflict between recognizing the need for reform and the (occasional) inability to press for it results in a difficult irony: Many of those who are most disabled and would most benefit from social change are often (not always) those least able to fight. That makes it tough for disabled people to cooperate on action for change.

Many years ago, when a group called ADAPT (which in those days stood for American Disabled for Accessible Public Transportation) staged protests in San Francisco, people were getting out of their wheelchairs and crawling onto cable cars at the Powell Street turnaround, a big tourist spot. The image was spectacular. I participated in some of that and ended up going to a rally in Union Square.

My model of a protest rally was formed from the things I saw in the 1960s—raucous, dangerous times. Contrast that with what I found in Union Square, where people with mikes and bullhorns were trying to get chants and songs going among a group of people, many of whom looked as if they'd been disabled their entire lives. Nobody had a voice. People had no power coming out of their mouths, literally. I, too, felt a lack of voice that day. Today, I think that we do have more of a voice, partially as a result of rallies such as the one I attended.

More recently I've been associated with many disabled people who are functioning at high levels in their professions. That fact alone can contribute only more force and power to the so-called Disability Movement. By excelling personally, we advance the movement. Simply by being in the world we make progress. In that way, for all of its inadequacies, the ADA has helped.

Today there's more likelihood of someone in a wheelchair getting into a restaurant, for example. I talked with a friend about this just a couple of days ago. In the past she could easily have been denied access, period. That's no longer the case. Now of course, you might need to decide if you want to insist on a comfortable table in a good location instead of being relegated to a spot near the kitchen door. Sometimes when all you want is a pleasant evening out, such things aren't worth the hassle. We have to choose our battles.

One thing we got from demonstrations and the ADA was the chance to focus on our lives more successfully. If we get to be seen more, if we get better educations and fuller employment, if people are forced to deal with us as more ordinary parts of the general population, then we'll impact the lives of nondisabled people significantly and things will change even more. Ultimately, The Movement, Crip Liberation, whatever you want to call it, is about liberating individuals, so we need to continue bringing to fruition the worthwhile things in our lives, all of the things, personally and professionally, that have to do with our autonomy. That's where our power comes from.

Although it doesn't work for me to be on the front lines right now, I need to emphasize that my position is not about negating the need for activism. I'd be the first to admit that without activism we would not have the ADA, for example, which has become a platform where we can stand to achieve more and better results. But I also believe that there's more than one way to contribute. If some of us can stuff envelopes, say, or make a financial contribution, well, that's not where the glory is, but by doing what we can in the way we can, we might be able to maintain our own lives and avoid the feelings of annihilation that public expressions of anger provoke in some of us.

I wish I could have been angry as a child. My childhood experience was: You should have this surgery, it will make you walk normally. You should have this physical therapy, it will make you feel better. I absorbed all of that as evidence that I'm *not* normal, that I'm wanting, that I'm something that needs fixing, and nothing more. My mother would say, "When you walk, put your left hand in your pocket, you'll walk straighter." I didn't have enough sense of self to reply that I needed to have that hand free for balance. Now, finally, I have enough of a sense of self to say, "Yes I am good enough. Fuck you." When I was a kid I always felt that I didn't measure up to my able-bodied older brother. Well, now I can say, "You know what? He didn't measure up as my older brother. I'm disappointed in him."

So many half-buried things in my life made me feel embarrassed and ashamed, gave me that "not good enough" feeling. At the end of my first year of college in 1967, I didn't want to go home. I wanted to stay in Milwaukee because I had just begun the process of coming out. The only last-minute job I could get was as a door-to-door salesman, selling potholders and dishtowels, all that kind of bullshit, for an organization called Disabled Products. In effect, I was selling my own disability. That was the part that made me embarrassed. But it was the first job I got on my own, so that part made me proud.

The job involved walking all day long, climbing people's front steps, having customers react to my disability. One woman said to me, "You don't look retarded." Another woman refused to talk to me until she saw me walk away from her door. Then she called me back. She was crying. She said, "Oh, I'm sorry. If I'd known you were like that I would have bought something. Here's a quarter." Somehow I made it through the summer and managed, just, to support myself for the first time. Talk about mixed messages.

Back in my hometown I had a friend who was six years older. I'd met him in orthopedic school. Dennis was significantly disabled with cerebral palsy. He could walk, but he looked like a windmill that was about to fly apart. Dogs would attack him because they thought that he was attacking them! He wanted to have a job, he wanted to be self-sufficient, but he never got the encouragement or experience to know how to do those things. After my summer-job "triumph," in my self-righteous way I said, "Dennis, I did it. You can do it, too." In the course of trying to help him, I talked to my brother, who got him an interview with his company. My brother let me know from the start that his reputation was on the line, that Dennis had better show up.

Well, guess what? Dennis didn't show up. He couldn't face what was ahead of him. He said "yes" all the time because he knew that's what people wanted to hear and because that's what he wanted to say. But I realize now he had no sense of self that was sufficient enough to make him feel he could accomplish anything. How could he, after all? He had been denied a full education and his parents had never encouraged him to make a place for himself in the world, because they didn't believe he could.

Well, here's the part I'm most deeply ashamed of: I had a conversation with Dennis in my car, telling him how disappointed I was at his failure to show. My brother had stuck his neck out, I had stuck my neck out. I had supported myself that summer, *he* should be able to do it, too. Should, should, should. And what I did to my friend that afternoon made him cry.

Dennis cried in front of me. I was a significant factor in making him feel annihilated. I hate myself for having done that to Dennis, but I'm glad I can recognize now what I did. I did it to him because it was done to me and that's all I knew how to do. I wasn't offering my friend Dennis a damn thing but my judgment.

Now, finally, I know that I have a responsibility to fulfill my own potential, not someone else's idea of what that might be. I have the right to not put myself out on the front lines, if I so choose, and the right not to feel guilty about it. If what we're all working for is a worthy goal, destroying ourselves in order to reach it can't be the right strategy.

A Wedding Celebration

J. Quinn Brisben

Erik von Schmetterling and Jimmy Schrode decided to get married the day they were jailed in San Francisco for taking part in a disability rights demonstration shortly before the 1992 general election. They are a Philadelphia couple, and the idea of solemnizing their relationship in the midst of the nation's most notorious nest of gays appealed to them. They were with hundreds of comrades from ADAPT, a militant disability rights organization whose acronym stands for American Disabled for Attendant Programs Today and before 1990 stood for American Disabled for Accessible Public Transportation. The founder of ADAPT, Wade Blank, who occupies approximately the same place in the struggle for disability rights as Martin Luther King does in the struggle for African-American civil rights, was an ordained Presbyterian minister who was happy to perform the ceremony.

ADAPT had a ballroom reserved for its convention doings in the Market Street hotel where Dashiell Hammett had once placed Casper Gutman and his gunsel in *The Maltese Falcon*. Erik rented a dinner jacket and Jimmy found some white satin from which he could improvise a gown and headdress. I told him that he looked like Maria Montez, and he was pleased. All of us were pleased that we had been released from custody in time for a good party. Earlier that day we had blocked traffic at the entrance to a hotel where the American Health Care Association (AHCA) was holding its convention. AHCA is a lobbying group for the nation's nursing home chains. ADAPT wants 25 percent of the money for long-term care, which now goes directly from the states to nursing homes, to be redirected to home attendant care. Home attendant care is much cheaper than incarceration in nursing homes and much more to the liking of the vast majority of disabled persons. The nursing home industry, however, has grown enormously rich on taxpayer money in recent decades and has great influence with its political and media friends.

Jimmy Schrode is an in-your-face kind of person, an immense man who dyes his hair a magenta shade that does not occur in nature. His taunts to the police as we were arrested that day were so sharp that I feared for his safety. Erik von Schmetterling is quieter, a gentle person who was a physician until his disabilities forced him to discontinue practice. He is deaf but an excellent lip reader and alert and active despite increasing immobility. Erik and Jimmy are a great team as well as a devoted couple, a great asset on the eleven ADAPT actions I have shared with them so far.

Our arrests were not bad, as arrests go. The police were thoroughly ashamed of themselves, full of stories of their own about friends and relatives they had had to commit to nursing homes when home attendant care would have been a better option. We were confined for a few hours on a pier with nothing taken from us, not even my cane, which arresting officers sometimes fear as a potentially dangerous weapon. I had no trouble making telephone calls to my wife, children, and grandchildren. We were issued citations for trespass charges (later dropped) and released on our own recognizance in plenty of time for the evening celebration highlighted by Erik and Jimmy's wedding.

As the 1992 presidential nominee of the Socialist Party, I was the warm-up act for the wedding. I reminded those present of the common struggles of all oppressed groups and ended by recommending that they regard the major political parties as Tallulah Bankhead regarded the bride and groom when she remarked, "I've had them both, and they're awful." Then I took my place to witness the wedding.

A disability rights group is a good wedding audience. Many persons confined to nursing homes are not allowed to marry, one of the reasons ADAPT fights for home attendant care. Abled persons are nearly always discouraged by their friends and relatives from marrying disabled persons, and disabled persons are discouraged from marrying each other and from having children, even when there is every expectation that such children will not share the disabilities of their parents. A wedding is a triumph in the disability community.

Every disability is unique, and the disabled have developed an awesome variety of techniques for satisfying their sexual needs. Some disabled share cultural prejudices with the abled, including homophobia, but this ADAPT group was clearly enjoying watching Erik and Jimmy declare their commitment to each other before friends.

My guest that evening, a San Francisco Socialist with AIDS, greatly enjoyed the ceremony. So did a friend seated near us, Irene Norwood. Irene is an African American from Chicago, a formidable woman who usually brings one of her nearly four dozen grandchildren to push her wheelchair during ADAPT actions. She is a pillar of a West Side church not noted for its tolerance of lesbians and gays, in the heart of a community where gay bashing is common. Yet she was clearly enjoying both the camp and the serious aspects of the ceremony.

Wade Blank knew why that was so and explained it to me later that evening: "The disabled and gays have something in common that they share with almost no other oppressed group: they are often rejected by their own families. Groups like ours become families."

That was the last conversation I ever had with Wade. He died in Mexico the following February while unsuccessfully trying to save his son from drowning.

ADAPT goes on. In November 1996, Erik, Jimmy, Irene, and I were together again at an ADAPT action in Atlanta, and over 100 of us were arrested. A pioneering group of gay/disabled activists attended that action. Irene died a few years later, but our ranks are always filled with good Baptist church women who know how to shout and love.

Erik and Jimmy are still a happy couple. Both Bill Clinton and Newt Gingrich double-crossed us on the bill now known as MiCASSA (Medicaid Community Attendant Services and Supports Act), which would fund home attendant care instead of nursing homes, but the bill has been referred to the Subcommittee on Health.

More than ever our struggle involves a community of interest between lesbians and gays and the disabled. All of us will be part of that struggle for economic justice that I have always called socialism.

My Dictionary on Dicks

Ed Gallagher

You are home and hear the weather's going to stay warm and dry, so you can get away with wearing lighter clothes. You didn't have a chance to roll to the gym today, so you do some shirtless sets of semi-aerobic calisthenics in your chair facing a mirror. Your upper body still hangs okay. From the chest up you are pleased. You contemplate what shirt highlights the muscle you've still got and which color best camouflages the bulge of your partial jellybelly that exasperates many spinal cord injured (SCI) guys like yourself. You wash your face and brush your yellow into whiteness and swish some Scope. You'll either shave or leave stubble, wondering which might better attract a handsome stranger to your lips. You choose the stubble because you think you're cuter and tougher that way. A little brushing, a little cologne, you're a cool hot cat ready to purr. Not for pussy.

You motorize your chair and look for a nearby sidewalk drain to empty the leg bag full of urine you're carrying because you know the club you're entering has a flat entrance but no accessible bathroom. You don't care if people look alarmed at your outdoor drainage habits. You handle this situation because you've done so before and because you have no choice. Besides, the club you're patronizing always has hot guys who'll put your mind elsewhere. You're probably not going to drink much anyway, for money and rotten bathroom reasons. Cool that it's happy hour time. You can get two-for-one and take your time downing whatever you choose. In case you do some light boozing, you've protected your digestive tract with a crusty cheese-and-tomato hero beforehand. *Salud.*

The bartender knows you. You make some chitchat and order a bottle of brew. You pay him and get back a token for your second drink. The club is nice at this hour, less smoky and less crowded, so you can maneuver around in your chair if you like. You do a little of that, then choose a strategic spot where you can watch who comes in.

Every few moments you wet your whistle with your tongue and peek at music videos blasting above the bar.

You drink slowly as more guys of all ages come through the door. Some are together and some are alone as they order their drinks and position themselves in other strategic locations. You think many are well-muscled and hot. But why in the hell do they smoke? Oh, well. Free will, free choices. You admire the way they look and move and tell yourself how forward, sexy, and successful you'd be if your precious body looked and moved the way it used to. You can't help but be tempted and tormented because you still think you look okay, but you know that your present-day body can no longer keep up with the sexual athletics that most of these guys are probably here for. You are not totally sure what *you* are here for.

After an hour or so, a nice-looking guy in his early thirties approaches. You've been eyeing him for awhile. Does he know? You could have rolled up to him yourself, but in the crowd it might not have been so smooth. And if he'd just been innocently looking your way, if he wasn't really interested, you would've lost the spot you secured. You're better prepared to meet eligible guys by staying in place, keeping your spot.

He is friendly and attractive and you enjoy talking to him. The inevitable "what happened" question comes soon enough and you give him the pat answer you've practiced and delivered a thousand times before. He is understanding and the look in his eyes tells you he has ideas of getting closer. You are pleased and ask him to pull up a stool next to you. For the next twenty minutes you drink a little and talk a lot. You are comfortable enough to relax things further by massaging his neck with your stronger hand. When you stop, he does the same to your neck and you know that the connection is happening.

He shyly asks about your sensation levels and what your sexual capabilities are like these days. You tell him things have changed a bit in that area, but that your mouth still possesses mysterious powers. Your direct and honest manner in this superficial smoky atmosphere stimulates him enough to make a play for your lips. You let him do this and return the action, going back and forth for a little while. French methods are welcome. You feel proud, almost a king among queens. Well, maybe a quing, anyway. You are not embarrassed about public affection because it is a gay bar and because there is really no other accessible place to spend further intimate time with him. You consider leading him somewhere seedy, but let that slide. He is a stranger, after all.

Maybe you don't even really like him that much, but the contact is nice. The moments count. You are hitting it off. Yeah, you like him. You exchange a final kiss and an embrace and he asks for your phone number or e-mail address. You look cooler and hotter by not requesting his. You keep some personal business cards handy for moments like these. Part of the balls game.

He walks out. Definitely cute. You think about what might happen if he calls. He said he wants to visit, but you never believe words like that in clubs like these. In a way, you don't want to see him again. You know what things will lead to at your apartment. How many times has it happened before? Still, you'll invite him if he calls. It is important to have those close experiences, especially for an SCI guy like you. You are a leader, after all. A terrific kisser with a mouth of gold. A prince in his prime.

Wow . . . some guys are hot . . . and sincere . . . at least for a time! He calls the next night and will be coming Friday evening. He goes on about your looks. You are flattered, excited, proud. But your cock does not share the feelings. You know in your heart and mind that problems lie ahead. Naked and in bed. While you're clutching chest to chest. When your dick ain't like the rest, will you pass the sexy test?

Hey, I'm a confident guy. But somehow, confidence in my sexuality still eludes me, even after experiences like the one above. It's unfair and superficial, I know. My penis doesn't agree, no matter how many times my mind shouts, "Every bit of sex doesn't have to come through your dick, dickhead!" My mind is right, too. I've had intimate contact "naked and in bed" with able-bodied guys a number of times. I'm older now, with C6-C7 SCI since 1985. (Screw coloring the multicolored beard I wear!! What's wrong with getting older, even among the pretty boys?) My sensation is very limited from the nipples down. My cock can erect, but mainly, the only way I feel it is via my own hand. It cums no more. How many of you boys with similar injuries can relate?

I love kissing and touching able-bodied guys. I enjoy being close with men who appear to feel likewise. But often I've felt like nothing more than the available catalyst to get them off. Nothing wrong with that. All in fun. All in recreation. But it can get old fast. Especially when my dong isn't participating.

Comparisons are useless, I know that. I've got to believe that this beautiful guy is in my bed because he finds me attractive. He asked me questions about "sexual capabilities" at the club, and I told him. He's here, right? Why do I persist in punishing myself for the things I can no longer do, instead of focusing on the qualities I have that magnetized this man to me in the first place? So he can shoot his wad and I can't. If I don't perform an intermittent cathing beforehand (a tremendously helpful practice, which I didn't do for years; ignorance on my part), I must delay the action periodically to put my recoiling cock into a plastic piss catcher. Maybe that's okay with him. Some guys like water sports; not me. Still, I can't believe he's content with the total scene, no matter what he tells me to the contrary. He might assume that I've gotten used to my bodily ways and that it's fine with me. But I haven't, and it's not. I've lost too much spontaneity to this injury. Too much time spent keeping guard with this injury.

Catheters, urinals, bed bags, and leg bags. Unromantic objects you can't hide away. The haunting truth persists. Ain't no doubt about it. I know how things used to feel. I know how they no longer feel.

This essay is not about despair. It's about levels of sexual frustration and the search for enhanced passion. Regret for sensations and abilities we no longer possess is human nature. But one can't stop there. It's also human nature to reach within to unleash the radiance, ability, and appeal we each have. If we choose to. I admit that I have some shallow perceptions on the subject of sex, dicks, and disability. Getting better, but still juvenile at times. What I'm doing here is simply—and complexly—laying them on the line. My truth, for what it's worth.

Sometimes I wonder if I'm becoming more inclined to dive into asexual waters, to see if my dick goes to sleep. But that's like drowning for many of us. Besides, there's always a fresh fish somewhere out there with your name on it. It's all in the bait, right? And the bait is the person behind the penis. I'm glad to spend time with an able-bodied guy and stimulate him. I really am. It's not that I get no excitement out of it. If I got zilch, I'd go out and cuddle some dog or cat. Yes, YES! I've had some nice times. But . . . (and, yeah, it's a big "but") . . . I've started to resent the orgasms they're getting, even though I'm happy to help. Am I crazy, selfish, jealous, or what?

C'mon, I'm only human. I can't help but remember angrily, wistfully, how my dong responded during similar erotic moments. How it responds no more. And how his does.

This has brought me to a decision. My ultimate sexual goal these days is not to secure some dude's coming cock in my mouth. Or elsewhere. My mind and actions may change, but I hope I'll stick to this path. Otherwise, I could live the rest of my life casually and restlessly, never jumping off this silly merry-go-round. Until I'm old and alone, that is—which by the way, is no death sentence. Don't get me wrong. I won't turn away a fling or two if the opportunity and mood arise. But I've got to draw a line, too. I need to believe that sex alone is not my main pursuit. What is? An excellent question, not easy to answer.

I think that I'm searching for a creative relationship where there's freedom from comparisons, competitions, and expectations. Fantasy world? I realize that I exert a lot of self-pressure here, but the flimsy gay games I've played seem based on looks and performance. And, yes, I'm often guilty of being a narcissistic contributor. It's high time to approach this sex situation more maturely. Now.

Two years after my injury, I started seeing guys. I had repressed most of my gay sexuality during my "walking years." So it was basically a new deal with me, a chance to be true to my desires during this second chance at life. Though self-conscious with my new role and roll, I found that many guys viewed me as attractive, despite the wheelchair. I craved that affectionate approval during those early years. I had to know that I still looked good enough. But that wasn't enough. I had to see if my actions were good enough. Not so much for them as for me.

My genital highs with able-bodied guys have been extremely one-sided. What I did to them they often didn't even attempt on me. When they did, there was no big orgasmic rush, anyway. Even in mental imagery. Realistically, I must conclude that I haven't had outright sex with any of them so much as sexual "activity." I guess it's the way I define sex. If I ain't coming, I ain't going. Probably a rough evaluation, but again, my truth. I realize I'm not being fair with this perception. It's wrong for me to define sex by the size of one's cock and what it can do, or can't do. Still, possessing one that can't do what I want it to do makes me feel that I'm missing out. Each experience with a coming man only reminds me more.

Yeah. I'm tired of being reminded.

So I look now to experiment with "my own type" of man. I've seen many handsome guys with SCI. I don't ask myself what their dicks can or can't do. I only know that I'd often like to move nearer, touch them more closely in intimate ways. Ways in which we understand each other's situation, where the obligation to explain isn't required, where there is no dominance or passivity, but a creative bonding and acceptance. Simple and strong. I've never had a potential SCI partner, but I'm interested. It could be quite cool—and very hot. Seeing a guy like that as gorgeous and vibrant could rejuvenate my sexual self-esteem. It could help me define sex differently. Maybe even help me cut down on personal dickheadedness.

And will this solve everything? Of course not, but it's a good move. Life is a big project to work on, not a problem to solve. I want to know that what I can give to another guy and get back from him is enough to create prolonged (even though compromised) excitement and satisfaction. For both of us. And, if that sexy goal is accomplished, perhaps we can breathe and kiss and touch—everywhere— a bit easier. We'll discover a more passionate and insightful definition of dicks and sex as we are. As we are in these chairs.

Four Poems

Chris Hewitt

REINCARNATION

In my next life I would choose to be
the mighty poplar—not because
of its great height, but because of its
heart-shaped, silver-backed leaves
whose mass comprises a swaying,
scintillating spire.

Then I could grow up
trusting that my limbs, flexed
under stress, would not break,
as my fragile bones do now.

I could grow up knowing that
to be vulnerable, to be sensitive
to every gust of wind is not weak
or unmanly but a sign of beauty,
and of strength.

SKIMMING

My favorite thing to do with my father on vacation
was skimming stones over the waves.
He could throw a stone so far it would become
invisible on the horizon seemingly miles away,
kissing a wave crest only a couple of times.
The trick was in the angle of the throw
like pocketing a snooker ball,
like a hole in one.

To me, skimming was his athletic prowess,
his climbing Mount Everest,
his running the Four-Minute Mile.
(I was good at it, too
though I couldn't throw as far.)

How fitting it was we did this—
it resembled our conversation—
always skimming the surface—
snatches of words,
never daring to speak
of my brittle bones, my tiny size,
the fact that I would never walk.

WHAT BRAINS ARE FOR

Even my head is brittle—
Sometimes it feels like an egg—
Soft-boiled with a crackable shell—
a dent or two
and the brains would spill out—
my precious brains
without which I used to be nothing
but which now I use to be
other than brainy—
I can think attractive,
I can talk sexy, flashing my lovely eyes
at a man and get his number;
better still, a wink
that says "You're cute."
and he's not editing;
he means all of me.

THE LIFTING TEAM

Recently in the hospital,
and in great pain
from broken bones
after an accident,
I had to be lifted:
bed to gurney, gurney to
x-ray table (brutally hard), table to chair.

Each time they sent for the Lifting Team:
Solomon, built like a football-player with
a wide smile, and Merwin, smaller, agile,
a savvy bird. Each time Solomon would say,
(seeing the tenseness of fear on my face),
"Don't worry, you'll be alright."
Indeed, their arms held me in a firm cocoon,
I never felt the slightest pain.

When in death's last delirium,
I shall call on the Lifting Team.
They will arrive as angels at my bedside,
and Solomon will say, "Don't worry, you'll be alright."
And they will halt my ghastly nosedive into hell,
and lift me up, up, high up
into the fields of stars.

On Being (Un)Representative:
In Memory of Barbara and Daniel

Danny Kodmur

Just over a year ago, I was hospitalized, not for the first time, and probably not for the last. I'm hardly a grizzled veteran of such places; unlike many other disabled people, I've spent many more hours watching medical shows on television than I have spent living the Patient Experience. Nevertheless, I know the drill.

So when a man was pushed in on a bed to be my roommate, I tried not to pay too much attention, to keep to myself. This detachment soon proved impossible, because his bed became the hardly calm center of a bitter, anguished hurricane. He kept screaming to the staff that he was in pain, that his history as a drug user meant he needed fifty times the recommended dosage of morphine in order to get any relief. The nurses refused to give him such massive amounts of pain-killers; his own doctor was unavailable, so he began accusing everyone of being sadists, Nazis, insensitive bastards who enjoyed seeing him suffer. This went on for several days and I soaked it up even as I tried to block it out.

Imperceptibly, as he got meaner and more unreasonable, I got sweeter, more apologetic, and gently cooperative with doctors and nurses. Had the proximity of the storm worn me down from my standard feistiness to a state of exhausted docility? Was I trying to be the Good Patient, as contrasted with the seemingly possessed Bad Patient in the next bed? Or was I just trying to score points with the cool female nurses and with one incredibly adorable, clearly gay, male nurse?

The short answer of course is Yes, to all of the above. But the real truth goes deeper. For the guy in the next bed wasn't just a furious paranoid drug addict; he was, in fact, another disabled guy and wheelchair user, who had used illegal drugs and prescription pills to dull the constant pain he had felt for many years from an incomplete spinal cord injury.

121

So I wasn't just separating good from bad, cooperative from paranoid. On a certain level, I was saying to the able-bodied hospital staffers, "Hey, look. We may both be in chairs, but he is not me, and I am not him." Perhaps I was doing this to set myself apart, out of fear of being lumped in with someone on the basis of a shared but not totally defining characteristic, but several months of introspection have persuaded me otherwise.

Let me take you on a voyage, transported by the Wayback Machine some of you may remember from old Mr. Peabody cartoons. Maybe some self-examination will show us all, me as well as you, why my life so far has been an awkward oscillation between being part of and being separate from the community of other people with disabilities.

When my parents started me at special ed school at age three, I began navigating my way: between adults and children, between the able-bodied world and the new world of disability opening up around me. Though I made friends readily with the other kids, I was already enough attuned to the rhythms of adult behavior that conversing with teachers and parents became normal for me. I don't think I was choosing sides; it's more that I was realizing what an educational community was, and that I liked knowing how it worked, enjoyed being in on the process.

Riding home on the bus every afternoon, my friend John and I would act out scenes from the cop and paramedic shows we were obsessed with. I don't remember making any allowances for us both being in wheelchairs, nor do I recall consciously inventing able-bodied personas for ourselves. We were just the characters, in ways that were both highly abstract and very concrete. When John got dropped off, the role-playing would stop and I would talk to another kid or to the bus driver. When I got dropped off, once someone helped get me and my wheelchair into the house, my disabled world would recede until the next morning when the bus's horn would honk and bring it back to life again.

At home, I was surrounded by my sister, her friends, and their friends from the neighborhood, some of whom would later become my friends. It was an able-bodied world, as enveloping and unconscious in its way as was the special ed school. I didn't realize how wide the split had become until several years went by, and my parents and teachers began considering sending me to my neighborhood elementary school.

I remember being excited. I loved the enriching multifaceted uniqueness of the special ed school, but I had been there seven years, and it was time for a fundamental change. Once my parents' fears and hesitations had been somewhat allayed, the period of transition began. Because the adults in charge were enlightened and because mainstreaming was new territory for all of us, I was treated as a full person rather than as the object of a social experiment. My parents had the final say at all stages, but I got a vote, and a chance to talk and to be heard. As a brainy, mouthy kid, I made the most of such opportunities, maybe more than I should have, but I couldn't help it. This was momentous change, this was process, this was politics, this was theater, and I was part of it.

The administrator in charge of mainstreaming used to tell me that I was, in a way, their test case, their Jackie Robinson. If the changeover went well for me, others would follow. If not, others might still emerge, but progress would be much slower and more careful. Like Jackie, I would be a symbol of change, a sign of a social transition that would be welcomed by some and feared by others. Like Jackie, I would need to be even better than anyone expected, and to be a quiet educator of others.

Well, stoic dignified endurance may have been prudent in baseball in 1947, but it didn't feel right in 1975, not for me. I had the sense that I was not some isolated pilgrim from another world but instead the initial scout for a full-scale benevolent invasion; I might be the first, but friends of mine, real people like John, would follow me into regular school. What I didn't count on, though, was that I would get caught up in trying to make able-bodied friends at a difficult age, in talking a lot to teachers and other adults about disability, in trying to figure out who I was. I didn't realize that developing my individuality would conflict with how I was seen and presented, as a symbolic figure, the abstract sole and legitimate representative of students with disabilities.

As I went through elementary school, junior high, and high school, I didn't have any disabled friends. I remember once my parents tried to get me to go to a teen group at the local cerebral palsy center. I hit the roof. They explained they wanted me to have some disabled friends. At the time, I was coping with all kinds of social awkwardness and disappointment trying to make able-bodied friends. I guess I felt that returning to the world of disabled people would be a defeat, like a courier bringing back dispiriting news from the scene of a distant battle.

Ironically, during this time, I worked hard on issues of disability access and inclusion and was an activist politically and symbolically. Even though I thought it ridiculous and sentimental to be given press coverage just for being disabled, I still enjoyed it and said yes to most of it. I served on committees, gave workshops, talks, and speeches, even made an educational video about my experiences. I got elected twice to school offices, and part of me remains proud of that, but I'm going to remember not going to the senior prom just as much as anything else. I realize now that working on disability issues was easy for me—a low-risk, high-reward way of confronting some problems while avoiding others. Work was recreation; just being disabled was and remains the hard part.

In these years the connection to my former life was tenuous, tense, difficult. My only links to my old school were with teachers and parents. I'd lost touch with John, my senior partner from the police station and rescue squad. The other two disabled kids my family and I were close to both died. I felt isolated from the world of my fellow students.

Much as I loved and honored them, the special ed teachers and parents couldn't really help me feel better. I couldn't name what I was feeling, and they had so much invested in me as both a surviving child and as the school's major success story that it all became part of the publicity machine. I wish I could be virtuous and say I barely tolerated it, that it disgusted me, but I loved being special and unique. The sadness and isolation I felt was buried under the accolades and the attention. All the positive spin helped me feel better about myself, but it continued to mark me as different and separate. I wondered where all the other disabled kids were, but in retrospect, I'm not sure I really wanted to know.

When the time came to go off to college, I had a choice between two Northern California schools. At one, I would have become part of a large and active disabled community, while at the other, I would become part of a tiny community that was still in the throes of diffusing itself throughout the campus. One campus would have meant being scooped up and lumped in with a group, while the other promised unique individual attention and a collaborative partnership with faculty and staff.

The prospect of being one of the few was more comforting and less frightening than the reality of facing up to a community, so my choice was made. The process of integrating an institution, of being a pioneer, was difficult, painful, even in some senses unnatural, but it was the devil I knew, the situation that was most challenging without being threatening. I knew I was well-suited for a particular, quiet kind of institutional politics; I'd managed to find a way of pushing a school or a community toward a goal without making them feel as if they were being held hostage.

I decided against Berkeley not because I thought of myself as an assimilationist who was now above the disabled world whence I'd come. Paradoxically, it was the reverse. I didn't feel that my mainstreamed life had helped me to retain credentials and credibility within the disabled world. I'd become far more adept at talking to able-bodied people. They may not have been my community, but they had been my audience, and in the language of vaudeville, I worked as a solo.

I worried that other disabled people, like my cousin Barbara, would expect me to stop playing nice and kick the asses that needed to be kicked. I worried I wasn't radical enough or fierce enough, that my ego had lulled me into thinking I'd been accomplishing things, when all I'd really done was sold out and lost sight of who I was. So I hid from Berkeley, hid from disabled identity, even as I became its quiet advocate in the councils of a much more tranquil place.

When the time came for my next school, I was all set to continue my pattern, as a less deluded, less solitary Quixote still tilting at windmills out in the able-bodied world. Thankfully, someone I respected sat down with me and told me it wasn't my job to break access barriers at yet another institution. He told me I needed to focus on me, on who I was, and what I wanted to do with my life; in effect, he gave me permission to retire from the Jackie Robinson business, and to make the life decision that was best for me. It is probably no accident, then, that I ended up at Berkeley, a place whose centrality in disabled life, culture, and politics had intimidated me for years.

Berkeley was and is thoroughly disability saturated, almost to the point of occasional inebriation or even toxicity. I quickly realized that the disabled universe there was too vast and rich for me to feel anything beyond confusion. I didn't have the immediate sense of home I'd been hoping to find, but the sense of independence and personal possibility Berkeley embodied enabled me to achieve several firsts, for once none of them fodder for the Pioneer Publicity Machine. First time buying anything in a store by myself, first night out to eat, first movie in a theater, and yes . . . even, my very patient readers, my first sexual experience. Ironically, the world-renowned disability mecca did not make me more comfortable with other disabled people, but it made me more at social ease with able-bodied people than I had been since I left that amazing special ed school at the age of ten.

Much of my life since coming to Berkeley fourteen years ago, and coming out shortly thereafter, has been focused more on my evolving gay identity than on my disabled one, but I have finally learned that disability's early and continuing impact on my life has been profound. By comparison, the ripple effect of being gay has been minor. Having disabled friends for the first time in many years has shown me that I can share things with them that able-bodied people don't understand nearly as easily or intensely; dealing with gay men has made me realize that my disability affects the perceptions and behavior of others more subtly and sometimes more destructively than I'd ever wanted to admit to myself before.

You'd think that I'd now be eager to seek out a social and political home among other people with disabilities. To some extent, I have, largely with my writing for an online magazine called *Bent.* Yet in many ways, I still feel lost and alienated, which makes me feel and do things I'm ashamed of. For example, I should be happy that other disabled people, younger than I am, are successful, educated, employed. I am happy . . . most of the time. I am of an earlier generation, and because I've hovered silently on the edges of the formal disability community for so long, most people have no sense of my self, my story, my track record. Do I expect these younger people to bow as I pass, write me effusive notes of thanks, help me get jobs that I can't seem to get? No, although such responses are gratifying to contemplate.

No, I really don't expect them to be any more grateful, compassionate, or supportive than I, alas, was in dealing with the disabled generation that came before me. And it would be unseemly for me to carry on about what I was accomplishing before they were born; I am far too young at thirty-six to bluster like some old soldier long retired from combat, too much involved in the present to carp in a curmudgeonly way about lack of respect for past efforts.

Perhaps if I felt more like a part of the community, I would be less likely to wince at the conduct of other disabled people, such as my roommate from the hospital, or others I get grouped with whose behavior makes me crazy. Were I truly part of the community, I could be more compassionate, see their lives from a more humane vantage point, not feel threatened or dragged down by them in any way.

But years of conditioning and experience have taken their toll. No matter how many disabled people I am close to, no matter how many of them I love and cherish, I am still the solitary pioneer and advocate, trying desperately to push events forward and change societal perceptions. I can talk about disability for hours, write about it cogently and movingly, explain it to the rest of the world, but I still don't really know how to live a complete and fulfilling life as someone with a disability. No amount of training or mentorship could prepare me for such a task, and I am not sure my experiences have taught me any lasting or productive lessons about it, either. I may at one point have been a Great Explainer, but talk is cheap; I may have enlightened or enriched others, but I myself am still confused.

This piece has not come easily to me, perhaps because I have finally faced some hard truths, perhaps because I have added to an unhelpful complex of myths while pretending to tell the truth. Am I just a superannuated former prodigy who has not yet figured out a way of being a grownup? A spoiled elitist out of touch with the difficult realities of being disabled? Or am I genuinely marooned, someone trained for a set of specific purposes who was so blinded by the joy of being a public talking head that I never learned how to be fully alive when no one was hearing or reading my words?

I am open to all these interpretations, and now, having broken my silence, I wonder how my shame and discomfort will resonate with you, my readers. Do I feel better for having gotten all this out in print? Definitely. Do I understand my strengths and flaws more fully now? Certainly. If I had that hospital stay to live over again, would I behave any differently toward my roommate, who demanded the only remedy he knew for a pain I couldn't understand? I am not sure, and that lack of compassion scares the hell out of me. Was this alienation what those who trained me had in mind when I began my transition into the larger world? I'd like to think that others sensed my rootlessness and frustration and tried to help, especially my cousin Barbara, but she and I never had that conversation.

Let it begin now, with you.

Alone in the Crowd

Robert Feinstein

The blind man sat in the hotel lobby on an uncomfortable bench. He tried to remember all the things his mother had drilled into him when he was a little boy, things that were important to sighted people, but had little meaning to him: "I must sit up straight, keep my hands down, my head up, but not too high, and above all, not rock," he told himself.

Like many of the congenitally blind, he had a tendency to rock back and forth, especially when he was under stress, or deep in thought. His mother would often remind him, in the strange German dialect she spoke, *"Sei ruhig!"* and he would immediately cease rocking.

He forced his mind to the present. He was in a gigantic hotel lobby for a gathering that included a cross-section of the gay population from all over the country. Some participants were thin, some were fat. Some were old, some were young. Supposedly, some were disabled, but mostly by old age. Many were alone, but some had partners. He knew he was one of two blind men there.

The noise in the lobby grew deafening. People talking, music from a bar, footsteps all around him. What should he do? How could he even begin to make sense of this gay crowd? Why didn't anyone approach him? Was it because he was too heavy? No, that couldn't be it: he'd been told that many "big guys" would be here. His age was right. He was fifty, about midrange. He knew that his shirt was "spiffy" because his sighted female reader had told him so the previous day.

He felt so taut and nervous that he was afraid he'd do something wrong, so he just sat there. Finally, someone approached. "What a beautiful dog. What's his name?" "His name is Harley," the blind man said. "Hi, Harley. You're a beautiful dog." "Do you have a dog?" the blind man asked, trying to keep the conversation going. "Yes, a Labrador" answered the voice that belonged to someone he could not see or otherwise sense. "Have a good afternoon!"

He heard steps walking away. What should he do? His mind began to wander. When someone who is congenitally blind cannot make sense of what's going on he cannot enjoy the "scenery," and that's what was happening to him now. As the noise grew more distracting his thoughts drifted to things that had given him pleasure in the past, to details that he suspected sighted people don't remember.

He heard the sound of Michelle Kwan's skates against the ice as she was warming up for her short program at the 1998 Olympics in Japan. The microphones had been well placed, so he could hear her execute the jump: the scraping of the blade against the ice as she took off, the thud of her landing. He liked those sounds so much! He could recall minute details of an even earlier Olympics, 1994. He was certain he was the only blind person who knew that during her long program Nancy Kerrigan had doubled her opening triple flip jump. This trivia gave him a momentary sense of superiority and confidence. He remembered classical music he had heard and enjoyed. He thought of a time in France when his room was filled with friends: five or six had come to visit him.

He heard the voice of his aunt talking to him in the German dialect she had used. She was telling him, as she had done often when she was alive, that a hungry boy had to eat what was on his plate. How he missed her. How he wished they could talk together in that strange, dying language. He caught himself rocking. *"Sei ruhig!"* he ordered.

Suddenly, here was "Wolfman," one of the gathering's organizers. "Come on," he urged, "I want to take you around to meet some people. They've heard all about you." The blind man got to his feet, took Wolfman's arm, and off they went. In a five-minute blur he was hugged and introduced to ten or more people. He knew he'd never recognize any of them, or have contact with these guys again in any meaningful way, but he went through the motions. He was overcome with a feeling of profound loneliness.

After the last hug, he excused himself and asked how to find the Camp Street exit. His dog needed to go out, he explained. Earlier, one of the men had helped him find a place for Harley. He couldn't help thinking, with some disgust, that that was about all the help he'd had the time to offer. "I'll go with you," offered Wolfman. "Thanks," he replied, "but I have to go alone, or Harley won't park . . . um . . . go to the bathroom." He'd slipped up and used the training school term, one he knew sighted people wouldn't understand. Harley found the single skinny potted tree and parked.

The blind man walked back into the hotel, but he knew that his dog wouldn't be able to find the elevators. "Can someone show me where the elevator is?" he called out. This was so hard. He had a master's degree in French, but he couldn't find a hotel elevator. He waited until someone offered to help. "I'm on the twenty-third floor," he said, "please take me to that bank of elevators." There were four, two on each side, far apart. He listened intently, hoping the one nearest him would open, but heard one of the others instead. Somehow he managed to push himself in without getting hit by the closing doors. He found his room and lay down on the bed.

He hadn't planned to sleep so long, but it was after eight when he woke up. "Where will I have dinner?" he asked his dog. Harley wagged, and he held him tight, petting him, and feeling his body from head to tail. Together, man and dog left their room. After finding the infamous Camp Street exit (amazing how many sighted people told him there was no such thing) and letting Harley park, he asked for the hotel dining room. Alone with his dog, he had his supper, then returned to the benches in the lobby. More questions about Harley, but mostly sitting and waiting. What was he waiting for? He didn't know. He knew he wanted to go home. But only one day had passed. Maybe things would get better tomorrow. They couldn't be any worse. At least Harley had parked.

When he was growing up, his mother had insisted that he was just like everyone else. "They see with their eyes," she'd say. "You see with your fingers; that's the only difference." He wondered what she would think if she could see him now.

The next morning he didn't feel like getting up, and stayed in bed until lunchtime. He had no one to have lunch with and he couldn't afford hotel prices, so he set out with Harley to find a restaurant. After asking some people, he was directed to a pleasant café. To get there, he and Harley had to cross a three-lane street. Luckily, someone helped them. But how would he get back across that street? Oh, well. No need worrying until he'd had his lunch.

After lunch he wanted to buy deodorant and some Life Savers, so he asked the cashier where to find a drugstore. An employee standing nearby offered to walk with him. He could tell from her voice that she was a black woman. It was seven blocks or so, but she walked next to him all the way, chatting amiably about the different stores they were passing, never once expressing impatience. He tried to make mental notes about where they were going, feeling more desperate by the minute. It was no use; he was lost. He didn't even know the address of the hotel, but he knew the name. It was the Sheraton, and yes, it was on Atlantic Avenue. Or was it Atlantic Street? Anyway, he'd worry about that later. They finally reached the drugstore. Nobody in New York would have been so helpful, he mused. Maybe I should move to New Orleans. People seem nicer, even if nobody wants to talk to me at the hotel. Maybe it's because I'm no good at doing gay things: maybe I'm not even a true gay person. After all, I don't like sucking cock. Maybe I'm asexual. Maybe it's all a big joke played on me by the universe. The woman's voice jolted him back to the present. "Are you all right? You aren't answering me." "Oh, I'm sorry. I guess I'm just tired." "Here's the drugstore," she said, and he thanked her for her help.

Inside, people were kind and he got what he needed. Someone helped him find that intimidating street and they crossed it together. After first going into the wrong hotel, he managed to find the right one. "Wow!" he said to Harley when they'd reached their room. "We did it. Good boy! We found a restaurant and we found a drugstore and we found the hotel and we're back in our room. You're a good dog, Harley."

After a nap, he called the other blind man he'd met and asked if they could have dinner together. "How are things going?" he asked. "Oh," Frank answered, "I had breakfast alone this morning, and I spent too much on lunch yesterday. I'm going to run out of money, but sure, let's have dinner. Wanna come to my room?"

He and Frank got naked and played around a bit. Then they remembered that there were welcoming speeches. They sat next to each other in the big ballroom. They listened to the speeches and tried talking to the other men at their table. The meal was buffet style, but people were kind and got them food. In his welcoming speech, Wolfman said, "If you don't get laid here, you might as well be straight." "At least Frank and I gave it a try," he thought.

The next day things seemed to be a bit better. More people asked about Harley, and an Australian gave him his room number. A seventy-five-year-old man wanted to get together. He almost said no, but decided to make the best of it. It wasn't pleasant. Neither of them came.

At the banquet that night, he was seated at a table of deaf men. Maybe the organizers figured all disabled people were identical. But one of the deaf guys had a hearing lover who helped out. Gee, he thought, here's somebody who learned sign language so he could be with his lover, yet nobody even talks to me. I don't understand. Maybe sign language is very beautiful. And maybe this guy is a great cocksucker. Maybe I should take lessons. He decided not to go to the dance after dinner. The music would be too loud, he couldn't dance, and besides, he was waiting for the Australian.

It was late when the Australian showed up. They hugged for a while and then he got the Australian off. "That was fantastic, mate," the guy said. "I've got to go now. Maybe I'll see you later." "But what about me?" he asked. "Not now, I have to see a friend."

"I gotta get out of here, Harley!" he yelled. "I don't care what it costs me. I'm having a horrible time. I was stupid to come. Why did I think I'd be included? Haven't fifty years of being blind taught me anything?"

He managed to get an airplane reservation for Sunday, so there was only Saturday to kill. In desperation, he called a blind friend in California, a woman named Toni. She had told him that she knew a gay guy in New Orleans. Toni called Ron, and Ron promised to meet him for lunch on Saturday. They went for a delicious lunch and enjoyed an afternoon in the French Quarter. For a while he forgot his misery and loneliness. Ron's offer to drive him to the airport the next day gave him a feeling of buoyancy.

After packing, he set out to find someone to help him check the room; he wanted to make sure he hadn't forgotten something. He had had the foresight to copy down a few people's room numbers in Braille. One man did stop and found that he had overlooked some underwear.

The next morning, before leaving for the airport, he had, like a grateful blind person, called to thank the organizers and tell them he was leaving early. Wolfman seemed annoyed. "There's a walking tour of New Orleans; I made arrangements for you to attend." "Thank you, but I need to get home." He knew no arrangements had been made. He knew that he'd probably have had to ask for help, and he was sick of that role. At home he could manage alone.

Back in his apartment, he flopped down on his bed, and tried to make sense of the past few days. His brain was spinning, refusing to focus. He felt as though he'd been having a nightmare. "A whole gathering of gay people, and I was alone," he thought. He understood better than ever the old adage about being alone in a crowd.

A week has passed and I am still trying to understand what went wrong at the convention. I know that everything the blind man recounted is true because I am that man. I chose to write in the third person in order to relate my feelings and thoughts in a more detached way. I felt as though I were two people: one trying to participate, another observing what was happening. What could I have done differently? Should I have been more insistent on being told exactly who would help me? Should I have explained my needs in a more detailed way? Maybe. But you can't force people to interact with you. In that department I really couldn't have done anything to change how I was perceived.

I've been thinking of the few people I've become acquainted with since getting my computer. Most wrote to me because of an article I published on the Web, and I answered a few ads on very specific e-mail lists, such as "The Chubs Digest."

I plan to place more ads, but I need to ask myself if my expectations are unreasonable: I want to make gay friends; I want a special buddy to take walks with, a friend who won't mind describing quiet passages in a movie. I think of my new friend, Donald, someone I met through the Web, and the wonderful walks we've taken together. Aren't there other Donalds in this sea of gay people? Maybe I need to remind myself to be as specific as possible about my desires and needs. That way, anyone who gets in touch with me will already have a good idea about what I am looking for. I will no longer try to participate in large group events like the one in New Orleans. I have finally accepted the hard reality that they don't work for me. They leave me feeling more alone, more isolated, and more unsure of myself than is good for me.

I'll admit that I have made plans to attend Convergence, a meeting for chubs and their admirers. Although this is the kind of meeting I just swore off, I think it's a reasonable exception: it will take place in Montreal, a city I like, and I'll make plans to get together with the few friends I know will be attending. This time, if I get bored or lonely, I can always go to my room and listen to French-language radio programs.

I will have absolutely no expectations.

No, that's not true. I am looking forward to being presented to the biggest guy there, and a friend has promised to help me find him. If we don't hit it off, I'll have a pizza with everything delivered to my room and revel in my debauchery. Who knows? Maybe, one day, I'll be the biggest guy at a Convergence meeting. Will that improve my popularity?

Love Is All Around:
My Life As a Married Crip

Thomas Metz

When I asked my husband's permission to write a personal essay about our married life he said, "Fine, just don't mention my laundry fetish." So that seems as good a place as any to start. My point is that I had to ask him where to draw the line. I've been an enthusiastic reader of personal essays more often than I have been a writer of them, so I'm not sure anymore what's appropriate. Am I telling you intimate details of my life because the confessional tone suits me, or because I have come to believe that bare-breasted disclosure is required by the genre, and I don't want to let you down?

I know that the only interesting bits of this piece are going to be the parts that either hubby or I find embarrassing. Why else would you be reading this? If you want to hear the party line on someone's marriage, you just ask your friends. You are reading this essay because you expect an idiosyncratic point of view and some searing honesty. I'll try to make this worth your while, but keep in mind I'm a Lutheran.

I like being married. I wasn't sure that I would. I was resolutely single for a very long time, not at all sure I wanted to change my single status. Naturally, this had a lot to do with being gay, a lot to do with being disabled, and a lot to do with being both gay and disabled.

I had assumed growing up that, if I reached adulthood and was really gay, if this was not just a phase, then I would live loveless and single for the rest of my life (which probably wouldn't be very long). This kind of thinking is probably very typical for a lot of young closeted gay people.

While in college, I developed a chronic inflammatory demyelinating polyneuropathy that slowly killed off most of my motor neurons. At twenty-four, when my disability became so bad that I could no longer take care of myself, I moved back into my parents' house. A brief single life was a foregone conclusion.

But life surprises. I recovered a small but crucial level of motor neuron function. I met this guy. My first running swipe at marriage was not a match made in heaven, but closer to earth, my second chakra. I loved Prem, but he and I were so different. When I met Prem, I was twenty-six and still lived in my parents' house. We weren't even officially dating then, but he was a "known homosexual" and my father's reaction was extreme. It set the tone for other members of my family. To this day, none of them has uttered Prem's name. I, who had been so puritanically literal in my truth-telling, began to lie about where I was going. I told my mom I was going to a friend's house. I wish I could take that back (Lutherans 1, Honesty 0).

Not born in this country, Prem was determined to succeed in the American way. I was pretty sure I was a socialist, and I wasn't at all sure I wanted to "succeed," whatever that meant. I campaigned door to door for liberal politicians, wrote articles for the tiny lefty newspaper in Columbus, staffed the AIDS hotline, distributed condoms in the bars, wrote press releases and edited newsletters, attended political meetings and workshops, raised funds, helped organize events, and marched for equal rights. If Prem had voted at all, it would have been Republican. He was studying for his radiology boards, totally stressed out, bingeing and purging on food, exercise, and me.

It was interesting the way things played out with Prem and my disability. He was gorgeous. I was a cripple. I was relieved to find out that he hated sports, nature, and activities that took place outdoors. I guess I figured if we stayed indoors, my disability would be less noticeable. The first time I went to his apartment building, I walked slowly through his plush doorman-attended lobby. I figured my jerky movements were less apparent that way. He was solicitous and kind, not the least bit condescending. I think he felt safe with me in some way analogous to how I felt safe with him. He gave every indication of finding me to be a sexy human being. I responded with irony and suspicion. We had sex, and then we split up, and then we had sex again, for two-and-a-half years.

By the time Prem and I broke up for good, I had moved out of my parents' house and was beginning to reconstruct a life. I was learning how to make a living as a disabled man who also happened to be gay, finding my way, successively, through the feminine world of textbook publishing, the macho world of the sports department of a daily newspaper (the losing team "got their fudge packed!"), and the strangely eunuch world of technical writing.

Fast forward to San Francisco. I was really on my own. I was "self-supporting," the sweetest words in the English language, and I didn't ever, ever, ever want to let anything jeopardize that independence.

At some point I became aware that my disability had intensified a natural tendency to subordinate my own needs to the needs of others—friends, family, or community organizations. My response to the social insecurity of disability was to work very hard to be needed. If I could make myself necessary to others, I could allay my fear of abandonment. I discovered books that addressed this issue and called it "codependency." It sounded like an embarrassing case of arrested development to me, and I worked on it. I learned to put my own needs first. I volunteered less, I learned to cook healthy food, and I balanced my checkbook for the first time in years. And I discovered that I liked it, the simple pleasures of a quiet life. I wasn't changing the world, but I liked coming and going as I pleased. I had a demanding job, a busy life, an expanding circle of friends, and more sex than I'd dreamed possible for a crippled fella.

Let's talk about sex, shall we? This was the weirdest thing. Walking down Castro Street, I felt both invisible and conspicuous. Invisible because no one cruised me and conspicuous because I was so different from everyone else. In the Castro I'm disabled first, gay second. I had been disabled for only nine years when I moved here, and I was still surprised on a regular basis by the sight of my own awkward gait reflected in the plate glass windows of Market Street storefronts. Surely that's not what I really look like. Perhaps this has happened to you.

Technology came to my rescue. If I hooked up with a guy on a 900 number, he never asked whether I was disabled. I guess it never occurred to him. Sometimes I'd describe the nature of my disability in very specific detail. Sometimes I wouldn't. I'd just recite the basics; brown hair, brown eyes, skinny (read "muscular atrophy"); and then we'd meet in a neutral location for a once-over. If we hit it off, we'd go to his place. We almost always ended up at his place. I think I have an advantage over other crips in that I'm ambulatory, and that fools them. They need a closer look to notice the extent of my disability, and by that time we're both naked and, well, a bird in the hand . . . (Lutherans 0, Sex 1).

But something still puzzles me. Why am I sexier if you talk to me on the phone first? Why does no one just cruise me on the street? I must be missing something.

At any rate, I found a method that worked, and screwing around was an important part of my personal growth. I'd like to encourage all you young cripples out there, even if your ultimate goal is blissful ironclad monogamy, don't shortchange this part of your development. You need to do it. I don't know why. You just do. Play safe. Try to behave with some integrity.

It wasn't free sex that made me slow to get married. I was reluctant to give up my own identity. I didn't want to become like the character Phyllis on *The Mary Tyler Moore Show,* who in her conversations with the perpetually single Mary and Rhoda, seemed to begin every exchange with a reference to her husband, Lars. Lars existed only off-screen, and in Phyllis's apostrophes to him. Phyllis brought him out, like a prop, whenever she needed a conversational advantage. She wielded Lars over Mary and Rhoda like an unseen bludgeon. Insecure and questioning her life choices, she must have needed that advantage when faced with single gals making a new kind of life for themselves. Not me. I was proud of being a single gal. Especially now that I was having sex.

But what if Lars is cute and kind and funny and smart and radical—and good company, to boot? You're not going to say "no," are you? His name was David. We both attended a right-on, mostly African-American church that featured gospel music and radical politics. We had both been founding members of the church's queer group, formed in response to the denomination's reactionary policies on gays in the church. David was queer, smart, lively, and he had body piercings, both seen and unseen. Very exotic in 1993. I love telling people that we met in church. After services one day I told him I was driving north for the afternoon, to hike through the coastal wildflowers on Point Reyes. He was charmed. So was I. We had a lovely drive.

Somehow that drive turned into a dating experience (exactly one month), and then we broke up, and then we started dating again two years later. And somehow the dating turned into a marriage. Don't ask me to explain how; I can't help you. It's partly availability and partly plain old luck.

Part of it is having some points in common for bonding, and something about David bonded with something about me. He is smart and kind and sweet and impatient and cross and fun and friendly and funny and imaginative and, politically, he's idealistic, outraged, and horrified (as any sensible person should be).

There was also the issue of safety, not to be discounted by a gun-shy crip. The disability issue had already been broached, seemingly against my will. As I explained to my therapist at the time, he'd already seen me fall down, and drop food. I think I first realized I liked him when we were eating in a restaurant and suddenly my hands started shaking. I usually prop my forearm against the table when I eat, and it's supposed to stay there to provide the leverage for lifting the fork, but on this night it had taken on a life of its own. Naturally it would happen when I most wanted to appear nonchalant. I don't know whether David noticed. He's polite enough that he wouldn't have drawn attention to it.

But I think mainly it was the company. My favorite thing in the world is to sit in the car with David and listen to our own babble as we daydream and stare at the scenery. I could listen to him spin theories for hours. He's smart. He reads *The Chronicle of Higher Education, Lingua Franca,* and *The New York Review of Books.* He can talk about anything, even Frank Zappa. He knew Mary Chapin Carpenter when she sang in the Washington, DC, hippie diner where David was a waitress. He cares about history. Gives a damn about politics. He has a picture of his mother with Eleanor Roosevelt and Jackie Kennedy. He reads aloud to me from Christopher Morley, Shirley Jackson, and the memoirs of second-tier Broadway actresses.

Shall we discuss sex again? David and I have been together for eight years this August, and we still do it. That's all you're getting out of me (Lutherans 1, Disclosure 0). Are we monogamous? I'm pretty sure we are. And I'm pretty sure I'm okay with that. I liked fucking around, and sometimes I think I wouldn't mind doing it again. When we first got together, the issue was one of limited time, emotion, and energy. I knew right away that there was something special happening here, and I didn't want to divide my attention. I wanted to invest it with this thing that was happening with David.

I have heard married friends, maybe most of them, say that an open relationship works, and intellectually I agree. But for some reason I'm reluctant. It's so mysterious, a relationship. It seems to work, but I don't know exactly how. I don't want to mess up the ecology of it. For want of further information, I guess I'm opting to keep things as they are for now and hope that whatever developmental milestones I'm missing by not finishing my fooling around phase will be offset by something else. Or maybe someday we'll make a mutual decision to screw around. Who knows? I'm not in a hurry.

Love and sex aside, there are practical advantages to being married, especially for cripples. As my friend Alan said, "I was OK being single, and I thought I would be single for the rest of my life. But I told a friend, 'Once in a while, I just wish someone else would go buy the milk.'" Right on. Do you know how much parking time I have saved in overcrowded San Francisco, because one of us can circle the block in the car while the other runs in to the store to return the rental video? Love means always having someone to say, "You park the car; I'll run in and save two seats."

But don't hope for the moon. My pal Mabel thinks it's funny that I married a man who can't use a hammer or a screwdriver. To me, it proves that God is a prankster. I said I wanted to be independent, right? I didn't want to marry someone who thought he had to take care of me, right? Mabel does most of our hammering for us.

And a husband can be limiting. David won't let me do certain things, like eat dinner out of the saucepan. He says it is barbaric and uncouth. He's out of town this weekend. I am cooking dinner as I write this. Tuna soup. It's something I invented from leftovers. Tuna, canned corn, and frozen spinach, with a dash of Mrs. Dash lemon spice. I am going to have to hide this essay from him.

On the other hand, if you do something embarrassing, your husband can bail you out. I couldn't decide which present to buy for a child and I was dithering hopelessly. Finally, I made my decision to buy a beautiful yellow moon-shaped rice paper lamp. When you turned on the light the rice paper turned into a glowing crescent-shaped happy face. Then I saw it had a rip in the rice paper. I bought a second-best present instead and went back out to the sidewalk where David was holding the dog. I sadly explained about the rip, and then I realized that I still wanted the lamp anyway. I thought maybe we could repair it ourselves.

I was really hung up on that lamp, thinking how a kid would really love a sweetly glowing night-light that looked like the man in the moon. But now after all the dithering, I was too embarrassed to go in and tell the man I had changed my mind yet again. Time for a reality check. "Do you think I'm being silly?" I asked hubby. "Yes," he said, without hesitation, "you are." And then he handed me the dog's leash and trundled in to buy me the lamp.

What keeps a marriage going? Beats me. Remember I said I was "proud of being a single gal?" Well, I'm the opposite of proud about this—I'm humble, for once. I don't know where this came from. I don't think David does either. It's just luck and happenstance. You're out there in the world, buzzing hither and thither, bouncing off other little atoms just like yourself, and then suddenly you bump against an atom you bond with, and the two of you form your own little molecule. My friend Alan was struck with the same dumb luck. Also resolutely single for years, one day almost against his will he bumped into Mr. Perfect For Him. Wisely, Alan observes, "I can't take any credit for this." Nor can I. I don't know where this came from or where it's going. Married people need to remember that. It could be gone tomorrow. Enjoy it today. Take a moment and say thank you.

The Boy I Used to Be

Raymond J. Aguilera

And that was the moment I knew something was . . . different.

He wasn't doing anything in particular, wasn't even aware that I was looking at him. He was just standing there, fresh from the shower, drying off with a towel. It wasn't particularly erotic, but I couldn't take my eyes off him, the way his arms flexed and bulged as he toweled off, the way tiny beads of water dripped down the back of his neck. If you saw him walking down the street, I doubt you'd call him "beautiful," but as he stood there, unselfconsciously, I couldn't help but think exactly that: He's beautiful. Weird moles, potbelly, and hairy back. Strange marks on his back and dents on his forehead only vaguely explained as the remnants of an abusive relationship. There he stood, rubbing lotion into the sandpaper heels that scratch the hell out of me and the one thing I wanted to say was, "You're beautiful, baby." And I couldn't. Does he ever look at me like that? Could I ever make him happy the way he was making me happy just then?

Do you have moments when your life seems like a bad TV movie? You know, the ones where the hero with the tragic flaw triumphs oh-so-predictably in the end? It was one of the first conversations we'd ever had, and I needed to bring the specter of my disability into the picture. Back then I was thinking of Michael as nothing more than a diversion, but I knew the issue would come up whether we had one date or fifty. My self-deprecation had already kicked in, so I dropped the bomb on the conversation. "And if I haven't scared you away already, I have a physical disability." To which he responded, "That's supposed to scare me away?"

I shoulda known then that my poor little heart was gonna be in trouble.

I told him about my cerebral palsy, my lack of balance, the fact that I was born two months premature. I made sure he understood that, for better or worse, none of this would ever change. What you see is what you get. He listened and nodded his head. A few days later we were talking and he casually mentioned a cerebral palsy factoid he'd picked up while researching CP on the Internet. I pictured him thinking about what I had said earlier and taking the time to find out more. I could barely repress the happy grin that was dying to come out.

So, what am I gonna do with this guy? He's adorable. He's smart. He's got good hair. He's a good cuddler. As far as I can tell, he's honest as a Boy Scout (more honest: at least he can admit he's gay). He's fun to talk to. Being near him makes me feel peaceful. Yet we could not be more different.

From what he's told me, school was a nightmare for him, whereas I'm the overeducated geekboy starting on a master's degree with no immediate real-world application. I always vowed I'd never date a smoker, but he burns through a pack a day. I get the feeling that academics (including me, by association) scare him. Owing to what sounds like some bad breakups, he's wary of anything that resembles a relationship. Sometimes, I want nothing more than to take him home with me and keep him there forever. When I see him, I'm happy. When he leaves, I'm sad. I don't know what I want from him right now, but it would be nice if I could call him my boyfriend. Even if it was only once.

Yet sometimes I find myself pulling away, and I can't quite figure out why. Have the sparks of attraction fizzled? Does the fact that I know what brand of toilet paper he buys—and that without his inhaler he snores like a goddamned lumberjack—mean that we've gotten too close? Have we descended from heady passion to the mundane level where he's just a guy and not the beautiful angel I think he might be? Or is it something more sinister? Am I falling in love with him and so afraid of that prospect that I have to push him away? For no good reason, I get suspicious and jealous and bitchy. When his cell phone rings I concoct fantastic stories about who's on the other end. If I find myself in the neighborhood of a bar I know he goes to, I scan the street for his car (all the while reassuring myself that I won't freak out if I see it parked outside).

He hasn't given me any reason not to trust him, but I find myself getting suspicious anyway.

So far, my friends all seem to like him. Last week four of us headed to San Francisco to see the indie-pop band of the moment. Michael had no idea what they sounded like, and judging by the Celine Dion in his CD collection, I wasn't sure this was the kind of band he'd appreciate. Still, his ability to roll with the punches is one of the things I like about him. We drank, we laughed, and eschewing any semblance of rock show cool, we danced. As the band ripped into an old funk song, we shook our moneymakers alongside the indie kids standing stoically in their natty thrift store sweaters. Yeah, we got our share of strange looks, but fuck 'em. We were having a good time.

Lately, we've even begun to express what I'm pretty sure is love (he doesn't say it as much as I'd like him to, but neither do I), and some of my fears have faded a bit. For one, I'm not so concerned about someone else swooping in and snatching him away. I'm not saying it couldn't happen, but things have come together for us, jelled a bit. I feel a lot more secure, and I think that's been positive for us both.

This weekend, we went to Reno to visit his family. Friday night we went out to the casinos and, for the first time, it happened. I had been able to avoid it so far. We'd talked about it, played out the scenarios, but it finally happened. It's true what they say: there is a first time for everything.

Walking down the street, la la la. I had a couple of beers in me, along with the happiness that comes with a weekend away. We're cruising along, and—BOOM—I trip on a crack in the sidewalk and hit the ground. All I could think of as I headed for the concrete was, Goddamn it! I made it this long, why now? I scrambled to my feet and looked around to see who else had witnessed my grand act of physical gracelessness.

"Oh my God! Are you OK?" Michael asked as he grabbed my arm. I gave a feeble sort of nod. Physically, I was fine. Emotionally, I was looking for a small, dark hole, someplace I could crawl into and die. He asked me again if I was OK. I told him I was fine, praying that it would magically become the truth. We walked a few more steps in that most terrible kind of silence before he stopped and turned to me.

"I know you're embarrassed and just want me to forget about it, but are you OK? Really? What about your hands?"

"I'm fine," I said, holding out my palms for him to see. They were stinging a bit, but other than my bruised pride, I hadn't sustained any damage. We walked along in awkward silence for a few minutes. I didn't know what to say. Aside from my embarrassment, I was fine, but what was he thinking?

At that moment, I was afraid to know *what* he was thinking.

I'm a very independent guy. I'm intelligent, I'm funny, and, thanks to the miracles of hair products, I daresay I am able to attract a decent share of admiring looks when I put in the effort to do so. All in all, a pretty good package, one I feel comfortable presenting to the world on most days. Then my disability reaches out and smacks me, just to make sure I don't forget what I really am, and all of that hard-won (and carefully crafted) confidence goes flying out the window.

Who was I kidding? Michael is handsome and strong and desirable. Then there's me, the helpless, clumsy cripboy who can't even manage to walk down the street without making a spectacle of himself. How could I ever hope to compete against all the other bodies that are so much closer to perfect than mine will ever be? Will I still be attractive to him after he's had to pick me up off the ground for the umpteenth time? Will he grow tired (or worse, ashamed) of my limp, my scuffed shoes, my scraped knees? I know that he worries about my physical safety. I can see it in his eyes as he scans ahead when we are walking together. Right now, I think he does it out of genuine concern, but will my disability end up a burden to him?

I tentatively reached out my hand and grabbed his thumb. I gave it a squeeze and he squeezed back, hard. The world seemed back on an even keel again.

Recently, we went dancing. He's not exactly the dancing type (although I have to admit that the Michael Shuffle is unbearably cute), but my birthday was just around the corner, so I played my trump card. After a few drinks, my gimpy ass was moving across the dance floor. I was having a good time, not caring that my lack of coordination was on vulgar public display. All of a sudden, Michael grabbed me and dragged me off the floor. He tried to cover up that guilty-little-boy gleam in his eye by swooping in for a kiss. "What's going on?" I asked.

"Nothing, baby," he said, pulling me close. He was selling, but I sure as hell wasn't buying. Tilting my head up, he started to come in for another kiss, but I held back just enough to let him know the jig was up. "Do you really want to know?" he asked reluctantly.

I nodded my head. I wasn't sure exactly what was up, but I knew something was.

"You were dancing right next to my ex."

Before he knew what happened I spun around and headed back toward the dance floor. I was dying to get a chance to size the guy up. I turned my head back and shot Michael a mischievous grin. The last thing I heard before the sounds of the dance floor drowned out his voice was "Ray . . . COME BACK HERE!"

Getting into the groove, I sidled up to the guy. OK . . . he's taller than me, but other than that, he seemed pretty unremarkable. I feigned getting lost in the music, bumped into him, muttered a quick apology, then found a spot where I could watch him through the mirror behind the bar. He obviously knew who I was, because I could see him pointing me out to the guy he was dancing with.

When I made my way back to the other end of the bar Michael looked at me tentatively. "Whatever . . ." I said, grinning from ear to ear. He followed as I pushed through the crowd back to the dance floor. Being the sore winner that I am, I danced up a storm to make sure that Mr. Ex saw us together. I even managed to look him dead in the eye once, before swooping in for the most passionate kiss I could muster while dancing at 130 beats per minute and simultaneously not spilling my beer. My relationship with Michael is not a contest, but at that moment I relished victory nonetheless. I was proud to show the world my prize. I poked Michael in the belly, beamed at him, and threw my hands in the air in a moment of exquisite happiness.

We're different people, from different places. That used to worry me a lot. Do we have enough in common? Can I hold his interest? Can he hold mine? Lately though, I've come to realize something: We *are* different people . . . and that's one of the things I enjoy about him. We learn from each other, and I think it's safe to say that we're open to each other's experiences. It's a pretty good bet that without Michael I wouldn't have gone flying through the Nevada desert on a dirt bike. But I did. And I loved every second of it. I probably wouldn't have had the courage to wear big-ass rhinestoned sunglasses to see Elton John in concert, belting out "Tiny Dancer" at the top of my lungs; I loved every second of that, too.

I think I've also opened his eyes a bit wider. The other night, we were snuggling and struggling with the fact that, no matter how hard we try, someone's arm gets smooshed in the middle. "My next boyfriend's gonna have only one arm," I teased, "that way this won't be such a pain in the ass."

"Babe," said Michael, "considering the circles you run with, that's definitely a possibility."

Homo on the Range

Walt Dudley

"Kiss me."

"Well, get your ass over here and I'll lay one on you."

"But, I just got comfortable on my brand-new sofa . . ."

"Jesus H., Walt, do I have to do everything for you? You're not that disabled. Don't be another whiney crip!"

"Oooh, Busdriver Bill, I knew you weren't one of those tight-ass politico correctos. Speaking of asses, how about getting that handsome heinie of yours over here!"

In fact, Busdriver Bill had already hauled his derriere 100 miles just to get here for our annual "Thanksmas," a Thanksgiving-Christmas feast, a little get-together for a few dozen friends, gay and lesbian, from all across the state. We even had some friends of Dorothy from as far away as Fargo, way out at the other end of nowhere. Either this Thanksmas shindig was very, very special, or said gay and lesbian friends were very, very desperate.

You may have heard that the Dakota prairie can be a desolate place—especially for queer folk, but maybe I should fill you in on the peculiarities of this peculiar locale. The small college town of Dickinson, North Dakota (pop. 18,000), lies two hours straight west of Bismarck, the state capital (pop. 50,000). The journey takes you over the grassy, rolling hills identical to the beautiful Dakota panorama seen just beyond young Lieutenant Dunbar's naked buns in the movie *Dances with Wolves,* filmed a mere eighty miles to the south. Do I mean to imply that prairie men are prone to have good-looking posteriors? Damn right I do.

A couple of hours out of Bismarck, after passing by several sad, depopulating villages, you'll happen on the next hint of civilization: Dickinson sports a state university inhabited by about 2,000 students. Presumably it's got its statistically correct share of gays and lesbians, but both town and college have closets in abundance, all tightly locked. Homophobia, denial, and malice are abundant, too. Relations

between us queer types are always covert out here on the prairie, so-
cially and certainly physically.

This particular Thanksmas, Bill accepted an invitation to be my
house guest—enthusiastically accepted. We had met two years earlier at Thanksmas. Even then I was in my new super-deluxe titanium
wheelchair. I'd of course pretended to be proud of it—but a wheelchair is a wheelchair. Still, the lean, Hollywood-handsome Bill must
have liked something he saw. Or was he playing some kind of game?

Without prompting, he told me that my multiple sclerosis didn't
bother him; he'd worked at a nursing home, he was "accustomed to
disabilities." Being mature forty-somethings, we made our first order
of business a discussion of procedure and protocol. Honestly, though
somewhat coyly, we talked of mustaches, which good-looking news-
caster was the "most likely to be," the fine art of fellatio and, of
course, the subject of responsible intimacy.

But back to the sofa: finally, Bill moseyed on over and we got
down to the business at hand. It seemed that our lighthearted banter
had gotten a rise out of our respective shorts. We quickly transferred
our feverish cuddling on the cushy sofa to a close investigation of the
plush new carpet below. And wouldn't you know it, my spastic legs
decided to join the party. Although distracted by my inability to participate gracefully, Bill achieved satisfaction. At least Bill did. Before
I knew it, we were hunkered down under a blanket and watching a
movie.

The following day we set off for the Thanksmas feast a mere seven
blocks away—in separate cars. That night Bill did not return home.
When I saw him at a poetry reading the next afternoon, I learned from
friends that Busdriver Bill, mightily drunk, had ended up at the local
Holiday Inn with a stranger who had wandered in from the other side
of the state. The next day when Bill came to collect his belongings,
we had another discussion, this one neither coy nor honest: "But, I
just got really, really drunk. I don't know *where* I stayed."

What does all this have to do with our investigating, or more specifically, not investigating, my new carpet? Who could know? What
does a titanium wheelchair have to do with just another one-night
stand? One may never know—only be suspicious. What I suspect,
though, what I fear, is that the Crip in the Chair is good enough for a
quickie, but nothing more. I get tired of the game called "who can do
the handsome dude in the wheelchair?" This here dude longs for

something more than a masturbatory roll on the cut-pile carpeting. I yearn for a real kemo sabe, an honest soul-to-soul, mind-to-mind, 'stache-to-'stache, and maybe-more connection. But out here in the Great Plains, the Buffalo Commons? Who am I kidding?

This tale of a passing fancy hardly gives a complete picture of romance in the Dakotas for boys of like mind and heart, much less similar boys of disability. Prewheelchair in Dakota, I had fallen in love, done some heartbreaking and had my own heart broken. But that was prewheelchair. Even then, homosexual contacts, social and physical, were few and far between. Is there something about Dakota, this particular sector of the great American outback, that leads to a gay-population vacuum? Could it be the general population void, plus the not-so-coincidental out-migration of the gay population to greener, friendlier pastures?

To complicate matters further, although North Dakota may be predominantly Lutheran and Roman Catholic, it certainly behaves Puritan, as does much of the Midwest—as does much of America, come to think of it. You won't find many Metropolitan Community Churches in this neck of the prairie, which is why gays and lesbians travel from across the state to Thanksmas—to find community.

When I was younger, I remember my mother offering that all-American maternal pitch aimed at every son determined to conquer the world: "Grow where you are planted." Years later I would write: "'Nord Dakodah'—as most old-country locals called it—land of my birth, land of endless, mindless prairies littered with buffalo memories, chaw-chewing cowboys and husky maidens, land I'd vowed never to return to, land of my rebirth."

My own piece of sociopsycho malarkey makes me wonder if "self-prophecy fulfilling itself" is more than just a clever axiom. Maybe all this vacant territory and fresh air really do something to the brain. After all, I did spend years running around the world singing for Jesus, herding the millions into the kingdom (okay, okay . . . I was a gospel-rock prima donna), finding the bright lights and back alleys of Hollywood, then adopting hometowns the likes of Los Angeles, Amsterdam, Honolulu, and Seattle. But now I'm back in little ol' Dickinson, North Dakota, thirty-five miles from the village where I grew up. No doubt about it, with all my arrogance, insecurities, talents, loneliness, doubts, and fears, along with my new titanium wheelchair, I'm home. With so few distractions at hand, maybe it's time to find answers to those questions about loneliness, disability, self-acceptance, time to find self-reconciliation.

And yet, all is not as melodramatic as it might sound. Just as with our annual Thanksmas, every Valentine's Day many of the same gays and lesbians gather for a public dance in the state capital, that city a hundred miles to the east where Busdriver Bill lives. I found that wheelchairs move very well on dance floors; lord knows, dancers always give a wheelchair dude wide berth. But Bill does not attend the Valentine's dances in Bismarck. He drives a school bus there, you see. Maybe he worries that the Lutheran-Roman-Catholic-Puritan school board members might frown on one of their bus drivers tripping the light fantastic with friends of Dorothy—a reference said school board members undoubtedly would not comprehend.

I haven't seen Busdriver Bill for the better part of two years. In fact, our sofa-to-carpet episode was the last time I fondled, nuzzled, and/or etceteraed with another man. However, last holiday season at Thanksmas, I suddenly found a cute nurse parked on my lap, begging for a birthday kiss. What could a wheelchair cowboy do? It was his birthday—and it was just a kiss.

Dancing Toward the Light

Bob Guter Interviews Thomas Metz
and Michael Perreault

Axis Dance Company, based in Oakland, California, has played a pivotal role in creating "integrated dance," a dance form designed around performers with and without disabilities. Bob Guter interviews Thomas Metz and Michael Perreault about their experience performing an Axis piece called "Hidden Histories/Visible Differences."

BOB: How did your involvement in "Hidden Histories" begin?

MICHAEL: I invited Tom to an Axis performance in 1994, where we saw some flyers for Axis dance classes. Tom and I looked at each other and I could tell we had the same idea simultaneously.

TOM: Yeah, we sort of dared each other: "I'll do it if you'll do it!"

BOB: Had your disability been part of your life for long by then?

MICHAEL: I've had polio since I was an infant.

TOM: In my junior year of college I developed what's called a chronic inflammatory demyelinating polyneuropathy that slowly killed off most of my motor neurons. I think I first approached disability the way I'd approached being gay. I looked at the social and political issues. But I was totally disconnected from my body. It was like, "Well, I'm disabled now; I don't have a body anymore. I just exist in my head." So when Michael and I went to that Axis show I totally freaked out!

BOB: Can you remember what aspect freaked you out?

TOM: A dancer named Uli, specifically. Uli Schmitz. People . . . ah . . . people racing around in their wheelchairs in a way that looked totally unsafe, that was bad enough, but Uli, in particular, flinging his body around, totally flipped me out. I seriously thought I was having some kind of anxiety attack. I thought I was going to be ill. I really thought I was going to have to get up and leave in the middle of the performance.

BOB: Did it make you feel afraid?

TOM: *Very* afraid!

BOB: Michael, was your reaction similar?

MICHAEL: Some of it I was expecting because I'd seen Axis before, but Uli blew me away.

BOB: One of you had better describe how Uli performs, or readers aren't going to understand your strong reactions.

MICHAEL: Like me, he's a polio survivor. Polio affected his legs, so they're very atrophied; he has no control over them. He uses braces to walk, but not in performance, as a rule. So that's the first thing I noticed. I identified with him. His legs looked like they were a puppet's legs with the strings cut. They flop. They move this way and that, depending on how his upper body pulls them along.

TOM: Another kind of disconnect, because his upper body is hugely muscular . . .

MICHAEL: That was the image that hit me in the solar plexus. To see his legs flop like that—in public, in performance—took me into my own shame and feeling of helplessness. I short-circuited inside. Uli was doing something that I'd always felt was forbidden. We're not supposed to put our disabled, imperfect bodies on display. The only public images I'd ever seen of anything similar were sideshows. But this was different. There was no prurience. It was affirming.

BOB: What made the difference?

MICHAEL: Here was somebody willing to show himself proudly in all his aspects. And people were willing to pay money to see it!

TOM: I think that's why I engaged with it intellectually, admired it. I'd been living in California for about four years and I'd seen a lot of performance art, so nothing was going to surprise me on that level. Queer Nation was active then, so I was accustomed to the idea that you could take the thing that people shame you about the most and put it out front. And it seemed Axis was doing that. The work was politically interesting to me and immediately impressed me as something I could get behind. And yet, what they were doing was primarily aesthetic rather than overtly political.

BOB: Isn't the artistic presentation of our imperfect bodies inherently political?

TOM: In a sense, yes. People stand in line, pay money, and sit down to watch something they'd maybe been conditioned to believe wasn't, couldn't be, art.

MICHAEL: Yes! The audience and the artists needed one another to make happen what happened.

BOB: Let's get back to you and Tom and the dance workshop. What happened next?

MICHAEL: We started going to classes almost immediately after that Berkeley performance, and that's when I left my body . . .

TOM: [laughter] That's when I said "hello!" to mine.

BOB: Are you saying the same thing in different ways? We'd better clarify what's going on.

MICHAEL: I "left my body" because so much of my life, growing up with a disability, was about the world putting barriers in my way— not only physical barriers, but social, attitudinal. We work so hard to break down those barriers—at least I think most of us have to— that we almost never reach the point of ourselves, being able to deal with our own personal disability stuff. If the Axis class had been just an ordinary dance class, there would have been too much for me to take on. I never would have been able to do it.

BOB: Was it an integrated class?

TOM: It was a pretty even mix, disabled and nondisabled. But we felt it was designed for us. There's no way I would have gone if it hadn't been.

MICHAEL: That's what I meant about barriers being in the way. Here, finally, was a situation where I didn't need to break down barriers in order to participate. Somebody had created a situation *without* barriers, where I could confront my body, my self. There was no-body coming at me saying, You can't do this. It was all my own shit that was surfacing, saying to me, Oh, you've never explored this aspect of your body, the possibly good part. Maybe you can do it. Now the possibility lies entirely within you . . .

BOB: How did that make you feel?

MICHAEL: Oh, I felt awful. Awful.

TOM: In class? You did?

MICHAEL: Oh, yes. I had no idea about what a dance class would be like, but most of the nondisabled people had had some experience, so at the beginning I felt like an outsider all over again. I didn't know about warm-up, I didn't know what those things they were wearing on their legs were. All that kind of stuff. People had their shoes off! All of a sudden I was a little kid again. I lost track of my own limits and I did take off my shoes, and my brace, even though I know it's not good for me to walk that way. I tried to fit in. That's so typical of what I feel in the world: that I've got to do the work to fit in.

BOB: Tom, were your feelings more positive from the start?

TOM: Yes. I took off my braces, too. I wear them out in the world for stability; I'd never think of walking around the street without them, I'd be afraid I'd trip. But in the dance studio I discovered that I didn't have to walk all the time. I could roll, or crawl, or scuttle across the floor. There were all these options that were open to me. And I also had memory of predisability.

When I started rolling and spinning, all that sort of thing, and moving across the floor freely, suddenly my body remembered all those ways of moving that I had not done for such a long time. When disability hit, my focus was on staying upright. Moving from one spot to another without falling. Here I felt free.

BOB: Was part of it the freedom not to feel ashamed, not to worry about "making a spectacle of yourself?"

TOM: That was part of it. I really did feel that this was a laboratory environment where I could experiment with movement. I didn't feel any of the sense of shame that I feel in the world. I didn't feel like I had to censor my movements, feel self-conscious. I was aware of how much I censor my movement at work, but in the studio I became aware of how much I censor it all the time.

BOB: You referred to a sense of shame . . .

TOM: Well, sure. I'd lived in San Francisco for about four years by then, and I was very much aware of walking down Castro Street and feeling like guys were looking at me because I was disabled—or else they weren't seeing me at all. It was wonderful to be in the studio and feel like I could play. On a purely physical level that was the wonderful thing . . . [delighted laughter from both Tom and Michael]

BOB: OK, you two. What's going on? Let us in on it!

TOM: Well, Axis develops choreography using something called contact improvisation. Things are developed out of natural words and gestures. You might come up with a common phrase, like "Oh, my," then find a movement that expresses that phrase, and then by following through on that movement, connecting it to another movement, it can become a dance movement. Or maybe you wave your arm in a certain way, then turn your shoulder and spin your whole body and roll over on the floor. It becomes about connection. And by doing this I reengaged with my body and remembered what it was capable of doing.

BOB: OK, but why was that so funny when you two looked at one another just now?

TOM: Because there can be a sexual element to it. And since I'd been in the process of coming out at around the time my disability first hit, the dance experience reengaged my body that way, too.

BOB: Do you mean that disability had put a damper on your sexuality?

TOM: Oh, yeah. Definitely. So after becoming so free with movement, I also became acquainted with the whole idea of, you know, going out and being free in the world. Screwing around. It was an awakening. It was a remarkable thing. I do not mean I was groping people in class! It was more a feeling I was able to take back into the rest of my life. The studio work helped me shed some inhibitions. I was able to say to myself, Oh, I'm a sexual being, too, and I can feel OK about acting on that knowledge.

MICHAEL: That didn't happen for me, although I did sometimes get an erotic charge when we worked on contact improv. I think that's because for so many disabled people the only touch we get is medical or therapeutic. I enjoyed the women's bodies as well. I was not used to touching women's bodies, especially disabled women's bodies.

Another difference between Tom's experience and mine has to do with his becoming disabled later in life. I never had a sense of, Oh, I'm back to this body freedom, because I never had had it to remember. So the rolling around, the "freedom," was terrifying to me. And then that made me ashamed because I was in my forties doing for the first time something that kids do when they're five. I didn't know my limits, I didn't know what to expect from other people. Disabled people just aren't socialized the same way.

TOM: Michael and I talked about all those things a lot, our similarities and differences, when we drove to class together.

MICHAEL: Sometimes we'd be walking out to the car after class and Tom would say something like, Wow, I feel so energized. I feel absolutely wonderful. While I'm thinking, Aw shit. Thank God this is over. I don't know if I can do it again. That's not to say it was a horrific experience for me. I was also liking it, I was also getting strokes. I think if I hadn't been doing it with Tom, though, I would not have been able to continue.

BOB: It sounds like you were coming at it from such different places. Could you really understand what the other person was feeling?

MICHAEL: Not totally. But I felt I was heard. I felt I was listened to.

TOM: Right. And that was more than enough because it was so much more than we were getting from the world at large. The workshop and talking about it with Michael helped me figure out what it means to be disabled. It's kind of like growing up gay. You don't grow up in a gay family. Well, you don't grow up in a disabled family, either—or a disabled church, or school, or anything. When you find another disabled person a lot of the communication involves learning about his reality. It's going to be the same but it's going to be different, too. So you learn about yourself from the similarities and the differences.

BOB: How did your dance class experience begin to move toward performing?

TOM: In May of 1994 we started classes and by the summer of 1995 we'd been invited to join a performance lab, just for students, that lasted about eight weeks. It culminated in a private performance in the studio, for invited guests. For me it was still about having fun, nothing more. Much later I realized that a lot of what became "Hidden Histories" was harvested from that lab experience.

BOB: Is it fair to say your lab experience was the bridge between class and performance?

MICHAEL: You know, I don't recall much of the lab experience, for some reason. What strikes me as the bridge was some of the verbal improvisation we did in class. I never felt at ease with the movement. Never. But I got a lot of reinforcement about the verbal stuff.

Tom, I think you did, too. The director would say, "You guys can talk. You're good." I think that even then she was looking ahead to incorporating some of our talk into "Hidden Histories," so we were providing an element that the company didn't have.

I remember one of the first times she asked people to do something like that. I talked about My Vacation from Hell, when my father died and I came out to my brother, all at the same time! It was a really hard thing, but I was putting out and everybody was laughing! [Tom is laughing now.] And I realized that I was talking and moving at the same time.

BOB: You were entertaining people by using the best comic material, your own pain. Did it give you a sense of power?

MICHAEL: It was the first time I felt adequate in that class. I had something to offer that somebody else wanted. The body stuff was so old and so deep that I would have needed to work for an hour to arrive at the same place everybody else reached in five minutes. It went too fast for me. With movement alone I was never emotionally present.

TOM: It was totally opposite for me. Remembering how I used to be able to move became about recovering those movements I could still use. If I did feel uncomfortable being physical, the discomfort vanished immediately with the joy of moving again. I managed to suppress the uncomfortable part in order to enjoy the good part. Despite our different feelings about all of this, what emerged finally was that we were both good talkers and the director eventually asked both of us to prepare monologues for what was still being called the "Hidden Histories Project."

BOB: By this point in the development of the piece were you just speakers?

TOM: Oh, no. We were fully integrated into the choreography. We had speaking parts, but we were pretty constantly in motion, too.

BOB: Michael, you described how powerful you felt when you began to develop your first verbal contributions. Tom, how did your monologue get started?

TOM: With one of those authentic movement exercises where you start out with a phrase that turns into a movement that turns into a dance. At one point I was paired with a partner in a situation where we had to tell a story. And I began to tell my partner, Jenny, the story of my hand: I can still shake hands, I can still hold hands, I should be glad I still have a hand. And then it became the story of my shoulder, and the story of my foot. The movements were all about shaking hands, and holding hands. I think that evolved into the story of the shoulder blades, and then somehow my grand-mother came into it and all those pieces got connected into the monologue.

It was really wonderful for me, because I had never documented that part of my life, never laid claim to that part of me. When the di-rector asked us to re-create some of that with an eye toward per-forming it, on the one hand it was flattering but on the other I had to let go of the idea that there was going to be an audience there. That would have made me totally self-conscious, freaked me out.

HIDDEN HISTORIES

Tom's Monologue

Shoulder blades: my grandmother called them wingbones. *Why they called wingbones, Grandma? Is that where angels grow wings? If you die and turn into a angel will you grow wings, Grandma, huh? Could you fly? If you die and grow wings could you fly? I wanna see the angels, Grandma.*

The history of my shoulder: I'm twenty-one years old and I have been a busboy, a janitor, a shipping clerk, a pallet jack driver, a grill cook, and I've worked eight summers on Grandma's farm. I mean, I know how to work.

I know how to put my shoulder to the wheel.

The history of my hands: my hands have been busy, too. But in the spring of my junior year at college, my right hand just quits. It stops working. It tries so hard. It tries to make a fist. It tries to open. I know I should be grateful. I still have a hand. I can still shake hands. I can hold hands. I think maybe it just got tired. I think maybe it just said, "Fuck you, Tom Metz, I quit. I need a rest." I think maybe it just went to sleep.

Psst. Waaaaake up.

Three and a half years later and a mysterious stranger called "peripheral motor neuropathy" has progressed through the rest of my body: it's in my arms and my legs now, and my body is never still. It twitches and cramps and trembles so badly sometimes I can't sleep. Neither hand works, and I write by holding a pen in my teeth. I've dropped out of grad school and moved back to Ohio where my folks can take care of me. Mom helps me dress. She makes my meals. She fills out a mountain of paperwork for the Social Security Administration.

But eventually, one day, things begin to turn around. I'm twenty-six years old and I regain some function in my right arm, my left hand, and my right thigh. I can dress myself. I learn how to write with my left hand. I cook my own meals now. I buy my own groceries. I HAVE A JOB. Life is great. But every now and then, every couple years— July of 1993, January of last year, maybe next month?— I get the cramps and odd tremors in a new spot, and I wonder what it means. Each time it happens I remember the last time it happened and I hope it doesn't mean now what it meant then. I hope it doesn't mean what I think it means. Something inside of me checking out, waving good-bye. Something traveling up my arm to my wingbone.

My wingbone, Grandma. Something's wrong. I don't see any fucking angels.

BOB: It sounds as if you both had complex reactions to creating your monologues because of where they came from in your personal histories. How did performing them, really performing them for a genuine audience, transform either the monologues or you?

MICHAEL: When I did an early version of mine in front of an audience (before the fully staged "Hidden Histories"), I felt absolutely terrified and shut down.

TOM: But Michael, you did it! And, as I recall, it was a huge hit, and everybody was shocked.

MICHAEL: I was either running on automatic or I was in a state of grace, because I have no idea how I got the words out. As the performance began, my shut-down feeling lifted slowly. I came to the realization that, Michael, you wouldn't have been asked to do this to fail. When my cue came to leave the audience and carry my stool on stage, I was totally calm and present. I just walked out on stage and started. There was nothing I did to make it happen. Or at least that's how it felt. I felt I'd done really well and the audience was clapping really hard. That was the easy part. Things started to get tough when it came time to rework the monologue for "Hidden Histories."

BOB: What made the difference?

MICHAEL: That first time I performed it the words just came pouring out . . .

HIDDEN HISTORIES

Michael's Monologue

[Enter carrying cane and stool] Heads up! I would like you to watch, to look, to listen. For starters, close your eyes. Listen to my footsteps . . . I have three of them . . . I have 50 percent more feet than some of you. Now watch me walk. What do you see?

[Set down stool and sit] Many people have told me I don't look fifty. No one has told me I don't look like a polio survivor! I had it when I was four and a half months old. Now, what polio often does is the same thing a drive-by shooting does. *[gesture and make sounds of automatic gunfire.]* Before you know it, little bits and pieces of you are gone for good. When I walk, I don't have much muscle up here *[points to thigh],* nor do I have much muscle down here *[points to lower leg].*

When I started kindergarten, my mother took me into the classroom for the first time to "sensitize the class." I had to pull up one pant leg *[pull up pant]* and then the other *[pull up other pant],* one at a time, so that all the kids had a chance to see my legs. I felt exposed, like a dissected frog. I didn't like it! I was wearing a full leg brace on my right leg and a half brace on my left. More chrome than a '57 Chevy!

So, there's not many times that I can honestly say I like being looked at. This is a rare occurrence. I'm inviting you in. Sometimes I'm looked at like I was the scene of an accident. Do you know how I feel about that? I don't like it. Not one bit! *[start walking]*

Keep looking. Help yourself. I want to get used to this too! When I was a teenager I only felt comfortable doing one thing in front of people. And that was dancing. I loved it. I was self-conscious, but my desire to dance was stronger than my desire to stay hidden.

You watched my butt just now, didn't you? Some people have said it's kind of cute. Notice how it swings. I have to throw my leg out in order to make that step. This is my bearing leg *[points to left leg]*. It bears all my weight with every step I take. It's the one that gets tired. My foot hurts right now. This one doesn't *[pointing to right leg]*. It's relieved of that responsibility.

When people stare, when they gawk, they don't know the history of me. They just assume my body is a wreck. So, go ahead, take a good look! What you see is what you get. And then some. Not many people look at me as if I'm a marvelous mechanism. They don't know that my body is a pretty nifty thing to be in. Hell, I didn't know that either for my first forty-odd years.

My hidden history is that my body is working rather well, considering what I've gone through. Many of us never get told how good our bodies really are. We each have a unique architecture of form, fit, and function. Visible differences? Yes, indeed. We have 'em by the pound. Hidden histories? We have them by the pound, too. We'd be happy to share. *[big smile]* Here's looking at you!

TOM: But then everything had to be solidified and scripted to fit into an evening-length performance, where we needed to create transitions around our pieces, so that they would fit into what came before and what came after. And by that time we were functioning under a great deal of pressure. We were working on the monologues in conjunction with all of the choreography.

MICHAEL: For me, all the issues of taking care of myself because of my disability went out the window. Here was a dance company full of disabled people, but we still had to do whatever it took to get the job done. At one point, the message we heard was: This is not therapy; this is not dress rehearsal; this is the real thing. This is not the place to bring all your other stuff. We need you to work.

BOB: It sounds as if what you resented at this point was being treated as a professional—very flattering—when you knew that, basically, you were not one.

TOM: In the classes the premise was: Come with what you have and work from where you are. For the performance, the definitions changed. The bar was raised. Which is understandable, because Axis is a professional company, after all. You stay until midnight rehearsing if that's what you have to do. And if you've worked ten hours that day at your job, well, you're going to work some more now. As a disabled person I've learned strategies for coping and I learned how to set limits in order to take care of myself, yet here I am in a disabled environment where I don't have the slack to do that because it's a professional environment, too.

BOB: What a fine irony. Here you are creating art about disability but finding that even here, disability impinges on what you can do . . .

TOM: It *was* ironic. And I think that Michael suffered more because his mobility is different from mine. Also, I was younger and had more stamina then.

BOB: Was there any difference for you between the demands of the choreography and the demands of the monologue?

TOM: I didn't really separate the monologue from the rest of the dance. For me, "Hidden Histories" was about both, equally. Even though it was often a strain, I enjoyed the performance aspect because I recollected the pleasure of doing theater in high school and college. I was comfortable with the idea of performing. But this was even better because it was a uniquely collaborative group exercise. I felt lucky to be a part of it. I remember one night when Michael and I were driving home, I said, "Oh, this is the biggest pain, it's so much work, I never want to do this again, and, I feel so lucky I can't believe it! How many people—how many disabled people—get a chance to do this?" We questioned whether it was worth it, but I know it's something I'll treasure forever.

MICHAEL: It's like giving birth.

TOM: And the other thing to remember is the special nature of the Axis audience. They're loyal, they love the company because it's unique and speaks to them in a way no other dance company does, or any arts enterprise does, period. So for me, I didn't feel it was my job to be a "performer" but to tell a story, to communicate, to bring something of my own to the table for this audience that I felt I knew.

That being said, I approached opening night with great trepidation! I can't believe I did this, but I invited every person I knew in San Francisco—for opening night, mind you! Remember, this is not like doing a play or something. It's extremely personal. Whenever I see a piece of performance art that's personal in that way, it treads a fine line between being authentic and being self-indulgent, stupid, and embarrassing. So I thought, OK, I haven't been able to see this from the audience perspective. I don't know what this really is. How good is our technique, how good is our staging? Is this going to be a wonderful gift to a receptive audience or is it going to be the most humiliating moment of my life?!

On opening night we were all in place behind the curtain, everybody lying or standing or sitting in the appropriate position to begin, and we're all whispering things like, "Well, do we have a full house?" Or, "How are you feeling? What's it going to be like tonight?" I was in a meditative space, reviewing my monologue, when I heard my friend Zoë laugh on the other side of the curtain and I thought, Oh my god, everybody I know is out there! My heart was beating so fast I thought: A person could die from this. But then the curtain opened and everything was wonderful.

BOB: And afterward? Did you feel you'd done yourself proud?

MICHAEL: I have no objectivity about "Hidden Histories." I have no idea about its artistic merit. I was gratified that I had done it, that I was able to do it, that I'd stuck with it. I was hoping for more of a personal transformation from it than I got.

BOB: What did you want that you failed to get?

MICHAEL: More confidence about being in my own body, although I think it gave me some of that. I was hoping it would reduce my feeling of self-consciousness in public. Oddly enough I did not feel self-conscious on stage, because I was representing a disabled man. But back on the street, with friends, with lovers in particular, I felt no different. I guess I wanted a conversion experience. I wanted to let the self-consciousness go, to be done with it. And that never happened.

BOB: Do you feel that since the performance there's been any long-term, cumulative effect on your self-awareness?

MICHAEL: Maybe so. After those performances, I became much more visible at work, I've had two promotions. What I had to do in performance I'm now much more capable of doing in life: being public. So it hasn't changed how I feel inside, but maybe it's changed my ability to perform.

TOM: I agree. There's constant discomfort and friction just living in the world as a disabled man. But there's another part of me that's adjusted—or become resigned. I wake up and say, "Look at this,

I'm disabled again today, just like yesterday." It's not like there's some guarantee that my experience in the world is going to be any happier or more successful, but I believe my response to the world is going to be more centered.

MICHAEL: I know what you mean, Tom, and it's valuable for me to have this interview taking place four years later. I realize now that I expected working with Axis would somehow lessen the impact of disability on my life. Taking part in the production really codified the impact of disability on my life. It proved to me that providing reasonable accommodation, improved access in the workplace or anywhere else, actually ups the ante. People think that access reduces the effect of disability. Well, it doesn't.

BOB: Access to the workplace is positive because it enables you to work, but then you have to go to work and do all those things that are so difficult to do because you're disabled!

MICHAEL: Right. As the world offers greater and greater access we come up against the reality of our own disabilities more forcefully. In some ways disability has protected me from a lot of "stuff" in the past that today I have to confront more often.

TOM: That's been a tricky balancing act for me at work. From time to time I've had to ask for accommodation, and it's been a horrible, wrenching, painful thing. I feel like it makes my disability more visible. Also, I'm afraid to be seen as someone who doesn't pull his weight. As far as possible, I avoid any mention of disability at work. I'll pin up flyers for Axis performances, but don't ask me about my own disability. Everywhere else I feel perfectly free to talk about it. But to me work is a performance environment, a place where I need to show up and hit my marks and I don't want to talk about anything else.

MICHAEL: That makes me sad . . .

TOM: Me, too.

MICHAEL: Because how are things ever going to change if we don't get to be ourselves everywhere we are?

Three Poems

Mark Moody

VIEW FROM THE INFUSION ROOM

The ridge of eucalyptus trees
rises up the hill, disappears
behind the hospital across the street.
Today it rains, the trees fading
into the low, heavy clouds.
Steam from a power plant rises,
its undulating grays
become a multi-storied chimera.
The endless bloom of this exotic flower
plays out before me, captive
of an infusion, seven floors up.

Steam: Madame Pele's breath,
the vents at Kilauea evidence
of her patient exhalation;
offense to her is no small thing.
Once, warned and foolish,
the end of a careless walk there
makes my current view familiar.
My breath was taken that time,
released in haughty languid billows
into a hot wet forest,
beyond a window like this one.

A whorl of steam blows toward the window
as the drugs wash through me now,
licking away like this memory does.
The nurse looks in,
checks the point that tethers us,
and I wonder about transgression,
remember that medicine is not forgiveness.

The rain on this colorless day continues,
it's steady tenor matching the drip
to the line in my arm.
I close my eyes, offering myself to Pele:
Please, allow the medicine to work.
Or take me up, like the steam,
that I might come over you,
mix with your breath,
and fall on your sloping mantle
as something good this time
and wanted.

PERSISTENCE, MEMORY

A handful of convex memory
now, that first time comes back
like the moment a curve of horn
peers cautiously out of the bush:
eight years old, the ball in front of me,
everyone behind, only kicking, running,
the grass tilting crazily from side to side,
my body bouncing on through a sliver of time
stretched into the languid presence
of a dream for which there was
no other world, no other feeling
than that of my little self—
an animal in its charge.

Time thickened
that way again, suddenly,
in an early morning one fall,
rail tracks in the dark street
refusing my tires, the bike and I leaning
into a slide, like an 'S' lying back for a nap.
How long that laying down took;
how much time to think about protecting
the new helmet. Enough time
for the voice to say, "Let the helmet
do its job," as the world tilted, curving gently
up to my left, the side of my knee
slowly abrading against the denim jeans.

Once, the doctor said, "Yes, I'm afraid you are,"
and I turned liquid, held together, it felt, by
a surface tension of the diagnosis I'd become.
The hot August world outside turned glass,

with sharp menacing edges at every turn,
and I stole though it, terrified that my skin
would peel back like a balloon at the slightest prick,
reducing me to a viscous, evaporating puddle,
billowed edges slowly shrinking
under the merciless eye of the sun.

In mirrors
an acronym stared back at me.
Lost in my own neighborhood,
I wandered while time curved
like a scimitar making strange
what I once knew, until I came
to a house that whispered my name,
opening its dark door to me. Lost
in its endless hallways ever since,
stepping over sloughed skins,
bones and ash, past the other undone
inhabitants, I've searched for a doorway
out into the solid world again,
where surely time was bending back,
until one day a reflection showed
that it was I that was starting to curve:
like the horizon of a distant memory,
like a stone caught in the surf.

MRS. ONG

Her skin is strong
and supple for her age,
the veins easy to see and find.
She's not really afraid of the pain,
but closes her eyes
and sucks in her breath
when the needle comes near.
She endures the stick
with a stiffened posture.

Later when the vein swells up
she rings her bell for the nurse.
"Too much blood," she says laughing,
pointing to the embolism,
"too much blood."

Yesterday's units have returned her color,
but maybe they gave too much.
She puffs out her cheeks
like she's been over-inflated,
her eyes a playful umlaut over the joke.
She shakes her head
as the nurse prepares a new needle.

All this fuss.

Later, the nurse tells me
that Mrs. Ong designed
and made the hat she wears,
and was once a famous designer in Peking.
She escaped China with her husband,
a famous movie director.

Now she lives in the Sunset,
comes up the hill for infusions
just like I do.

Today we sat together,
reduced to being patient
with our suffering, ringing bells
about our needs.
I silently agree with her:
it's not the pain people are afraid of,
but the idea of it.
It's not the blood,
it's getting too much.

Becoming Daddy's Boy

J. Douglas George

1.

All my life, I've never been the type to pick someone up.

I've never gone home with a guy I met at a party or picked up in a bar. I've never been on a blind date. If you want to get technical about it, I've never really even asked anyone out on a date. I'd like to tell you that I've done those things, but the truth is, I never have.

Cruising just isn't my style. OK, let's be honest here . . . I'm among friends, right? As a man with a visible disability, the singles scene doesn't work for me. When I manage to make my way into a bar, everyone notices my crippled body and immediately removes me from the pool of potential mates. Actually, that's a polite way of putting it. Let's not beat around the bush. Guys generally look right through me while scanning the room.

That said, it's no surprise that my dating successes are due to The Conversion. It works like this: I meet someone, we become friends. If the chemistry is there, we may become lovers after many nights spent hanging out and wallowing in the built-up sexual tension. All of the serious relationships in my life are a result of The Conversion. Sure, it's great for the heart, since a lot of rejection is headed off at the pass, but it isn't so great when I count the friends I've lost when the sexual relationship goes awry. It's not that their numbers are great, it's just that the voids they have left are large, and can never be filled by anyone else.

Lately, my romantic life has been uninteresting. One evening, with all my friends out gallivanting, I was home and lonely. I began perusing some online personals. OK, I'll admit it, I'm a big personals junkie. I always read them. I'm never looking to answer any, mind you. I just feel like they make good, sleazy reading. I logged on to an Internet personals site and started reading the ads. I'm not sure why, but I've always had a thing for older guys. Middle-aged men, with their graying hair, wise old eyes, and their soft potbellies have always turned me on. I'm sure Freud could have a field day with that, but frankly, I don't give a fuck. I'm past the stage in my life where I wonder why I like what I like. I just chalk it up to a lifetime of dealing with my own nonstandard-issue body that makes me appreciate these guys.

I'm not looking for a father. I have one of those. It's just something about middle-aged men, with their weathered faces and road-tested physiques, that gets me going. So what if they don't fit into any of the clothes at Armani Exchange? Sometimes a cashmere sweater looks better in a ball on the floor anyway. If I want a stick figure, I'll draw one. Give me a man with some meat on his bones, and something behind those eyes other than an afternoon of working out at Gold's. Clicking away at the online personals ("Gym-toned GWM seeks buff bottom . . ."), one of the ads made me stop and take notice: "Fifty-ish man, musician, seeks younger . . ."

Reading the rest of the ad, my head began swimming. I imagined myself curled up on the couch while the ideal man I'd just invented serenaded me. He also made sure that my wine glass stayed full. He would periodically pause in his playing, scrunching his face at something that wasn't coming together quite right. Or maybe he'd stop to ask me about books, or tell me a humorous anecdote about something that happened earlier that day, or maybe he'd ask to hear the latest from my in-progress novel. He'd offer small critiques, but mostly just look at me admiringly, eyes crinkling around the edges, and praise my well-honed vocabulary and overall brilliance.

The ad was wordy, a little dorky even. And I loved it. He talked of music and wine and good food. Conversation and cuddling and romance. Amid a sea of "8.5-inch uncut manmeat" and "hot, hungry holes ready for action" I had found an oasis of intellectual calm. Now before you go off thinking I'm a saint, above all the pleasures of the flesh, let me make something clear. I like sex as much as the next guy. In fact, probably more. You might not be able to tell by looking at me, but given the right set of circumstances, I can be a demon in the sack. Still, if you really want to get me all hot and bothered, talk to me. Use words such as obsequious and sartorial and mellifluous. Teach me about philosophy, whisper some poetry in my car (it better not be Walt Whitman. Sure, he was a great poet, but that's like sending red roses on Valentine's Day, or taking me to dinner and a movie).

If you want to impress me, you've got to be creative—canned-ham Hallmark sentiments aren't gonna do it. Read me Bukowski and Crane, tell me about the Discovery Channel show about the construction of the New York subway, or the dream you had about drinking bourbon with Hunter S. Thompson, dressed in matching white suits and fedoras. These are the ways to get me into bed, not bullshit braggadocio about your eight and a half inches. Besides, what good does 8.5 do if you last only a minute and a half anyway? All that blood is better off feeding your brain. Big brains win over big dicks every time.

I hit reply . . . and answered my first personals ad. I told him I liked his ad, and that I thought we had a lot of the same things in common. I mentioned that I wasn't looking for a quickie, that I'd rather get to know him and take it from there. I gave him my instant messenger nickname, and wished him a good night. I clicked the "send" button, and immediately freaked out.

I had never done anything like this before. Once the panic subsided, all I felt was good. And hopeful. I hadn't ever anticipated answering an ad. I used to think of personals (and the people who used them) as being kind of seedy. Still, the real world has proven to be a disappointment to me in that arena, so what the hell? At least over the Internet, my disability wouldn't be an immediate disqualifier. Still, I had to wonder if disclosure via e-mail would be any better.

2.

A few hours later, my computer dinged. He was sending me a message!

"Hi!" he said.

"Hi!" I replied.

"How are you?" he typed.

"OK. You?" I responded.

"Thanks for answering my ad," he said.

"Sure," I replied.

OK, so we didn't get off to a great start, conversationally. What the fuck do you say to someone you've never met, someone you can't even see? After five minutes of awkward chitchat, he asked me what I did for a living. He didn't ask about my cock, or if I was top or bottom, or if I wanted to party tonight. He asked me what I did for a living.

We talked about work, and books, and what kinds of movies we liked. Half an hour later, he asked for my stats. I gave him the rundown, age, height, weight, body type, hair color, eye color. At the end, I hesitatingly added "HIV negative." I didn't want to seem like I was hunting for sex.

"52/5'10"/165/grey/green/negative," he replied. Then, a pause, and . . . "9"."

N I N E I N C H E S?! My mind reeled at the prospect—and I immediately got a raging hard-on.

"Are you REALLY 9"?" I typed.

"Yes," he replied.

I reminded him that I wasn't looking for a quickie, and was really more interested in becoming friends first. We spent the next two hours chatting, about work, film, food, and just about everything except sex. I was up-front about my disability and he said he didn't mind. He told me about a blind friend of his at the university, and about playing the cello. About 1:30 in the morning he wished me sweet dreams and logged off. A perfect gentleman. I went to bed. Happy.

Over the next several days, we spent hours chatting. He told me about his day job, and about playing the cello. We talked about movies, computers, baseball, cooking. I explained my disability to him, and he told me about the partner he broke up with two years ago. We talked about everything. He'd ask me how my day went at work, and told me about his plans for the weekend. It seemed weird, but after a few weeks of these nightly chats, I began to think of him as my friend. We had still never met. We also never talked about sex.

One Saturday afternoon I got a message from him: "Would you like to come over?" I typed, "Sure," then hesitated before I hit the "send" button. It wasn't that I didn't want to meet him. I had spent many nights fantasizing about what our meeting would be like. Invariably in my fantasy he'd be handsome and rugged and gentle; I'd be witty and engaging. And I wouldn't trip on the carpet. Then, overcome by passion, he'd throw me down on the couch, lustily unbutton my shirt, kiss my chest, and work his way down from there.

I was scared. In the masturbatory fantasies that I'd cooked up, everything was perfect. The lights were low, conversation was deep, the wine was expensive, the sex was endless and explosive. Could real life *ever* measure up? When I got to his building I hesitated, then screwed up my courage and punched his number into the intercom. Next thing I know I'm standing outside his door and knocking and I'm thinking, "fuck, fuck, fuck, fuck . . . fuck." He answered the door and we saw each other for the first time.

3.

"Hello," he said, ushering me in.

I sat down on the couch, nervous. He sat on another couch, perpendicular. Then, he got up. "Can I get you something to drink?" he asked. "Water, orange juice, some tea? I don't drink alcohol, so I can't offer you anything harder." Well, so much for that bottomless wineglass fantasy, I thought. Feeling the chalky dry-mouth brought on by the worst case of nerves I've ever had, I asked for a glass of water. He returned from the kitchen, carrying two glasses of water. He fastidiously set each on a coaster atop the small wooden table next to the sofa. Having rarely used a coaster in my life, I giggled at his fussiness. It seemed oddly . . . cute.

We sat talking for the next two and a half hours. The conversation was decidedly nonsexual and he kept a gentlemanly distance over on his couch. Once, as we simultaneously reached for our water glasses, our hands brushed against each other. He blushed and seemed genuinely embarrassed. Still, as it became clearer that we enjoyed each other's company, I began to get antsy about what else we might enjoy together.

His voice was low and scratchy and mesmerizing. I also couldn't help but steal glances at the bulge in his black corduroy trousers. Once, he caught me scamming on the package and gave me a little wink. Finally, I crossed the line. I asked him why he liked younger men. He looked at me and asked why I liked older ones. We both laughed and called it a draw. He asked me if I felt comfortable and if I wanted to sit next to him. It was an awkward gesture and it made me laugh. It seemed so . . . so . . . third grade. I sat down next to him. He put his arm around me for an instant, then immediately retracted it. "Don't laugh at me," he said. "It's been a long time since I've done this." Then he smiled, and I melted.

He tentatively put his arm around me again. I shifted slightly, moving infinitesimally closer to him as a sign of approval. He leaned his head on my shoulder and we sat like that for several minutes, silent, listening to each other breathe. I turned toward him, and placed my hand on his chest. He seemed to like that, and pulled me a little closer. I slowly ran my hand over his firm chest. I moved down, and rested my hand on his belly, over his navel. I felt the muscles in his stomach tighten as he tried to suck in his small gut. "Relax," I said. I began rubbing his belly and he started to stroke the back of my neck with the hand that had been resting on my shoulder. He relaxed. I relaxed.

Then I reached under his red T-shirt and ran my hands through the thick hair on his chest. His breathing became a little more pronounced, and as I rubbed his chest, his nipples stiffened. I asked him to take off the shirt, which he did. He unbuttoned my shirt, slowly, staring me in the eye all the while. When he got to the last button, which was over my lap, he gave my cock a squeeze through my jeans. He slipped the shirt off, and in doing so, ran his large hands slowly down the length of my arms. He leaned over and kissed me lightly, right in the center of my chest. Slowly, he worked his way down, kissing my chest, sliding off the couch and onto the floor as he got lower and lower. He kneeled on the floor in front of me and pulled me forward to the edge of the couch. He leaned down and kissed my belly while he started unbuckling my belt. As soon as I heard the clink of the belt buckle, the fabric-metal pop as he unbuttoned my jeans, I got rock hard. He eased his hands into the waistband of my jeans and squeezed my ass. In one smooth, slow move, he pulled my jeans and underwear down to my ankles.

As he did this, he continued staring me in the eye. "Are you OK?" he asked. "Yes," I replied. He placed his hands on my knees, and spread my legs apart a bit. He looked up at me again, smiled, and leaning forward, took my dick into his mouth. He continued staring up at me, looking at once vulnerable and powerful. He held the head of my cock there for a moment, looking up at me with those green eyes. Then, he wrapped his left hand around the base of my dick and began slowly bobbing forward and back, teasing the head with his tongue. My instinct was to throw my head back and relax, but instead I watched him. As he settled into a slow rhythm he tilted his head to the right a bit, with an idyllic expression on his face, eyes closed. It was hard to tell, but it looked as if he was smiling.

He opened his eyes again, and stared me down. As he sucked and licked and stroked me, he continued to look me dead in the eye. As he played with my cock, he found what I liked and returned to those spots repeatedly. Stamina has long been one of my best assets, something that more than a few partners have expressed their appreciation of. As Philip knelt there before me, however, my stamina was beaten into submission by his superior talents. After only a few minutes, I felt myself getting dangerously close to climax. I was close enough that I knew if I relaxed a bit more, I could let him take control of my body, and just enjoy the orgasm. The thought of this delicious pleasure that I was being treated to coming to an end was the only thing that kept me from grabbing him by the back of the head and pumping deep into his throat.

He stopped. He got up and sat down next to me, pulling my head down on his bare, hairy chest. I was breathing heavily. "Shhhhh . . ." he whispered, as he stroked my hair. "Relax, I'll take care of you." He stood again, and gently set my head down on the couch. I leaned forward a bit, and began to open my eyes, to see what he was doing. He was looking down at me, straight in the eyes. "No," he said. "Lie back, close your eyes, relax . . ." I felt him untying my shoes, and slipping them off slowly. He pulled off my socks and then gingerly picked up each of my feet and pulled my legs out of my jeans. I was utterly naked, the ecstasy of sex still coursing through my veins, my energy level almost totally sapped. He fiddled around for a few minutes, then I felt him sit back down. I opened my eyes and saw that he had taken my clothes and folded them, placing them in a neat pile on the armchair across the room. He put his head on my shoulder.

Again, I tried to move. "No . . ." he whispered, "just lie back, and let Daddy take care of you." I turned and looked him in the eyes, his face a few inches from mine. We stared at each other for what seemed like an eternity. "Are you OK?" he asked. "Uh, yeah, I just never . . . is that why you like younger guys? You like to play Daddy?" "Does that scare you?" he asked. "No . . . I trust you. I . . . uhhh . . . it's just new to me," I replied.

I told him that I had never gotten into any sort of role-playing before. I also told him that I was afraid I would laugh, cynic that I am, and ruin his fantasy. He explained to me that his Daddy fantasies were only part of the reason that he was attracted to me, and that I didn't have to play if I didn't want to. He asked if I would mind if he got more aggressive (I didn't mind) and assured me that we could stop at any time. I stared at him, for a long time. He sat there quietly, while I stared him down.

On one hand, I was intrigued, but on the other hand, I was sure I would fuck the whole thing up. I've never been much of an actor, and just the thought of calling someone "Daddy" made me want to laugh. A small part of me was scared, too. Not of him, but of the unknown. I'd never done anything like this before. Would I hate it or, scarier still—would I love it?

He just sat there, holding my hand, rubbing my palm with his thumb as I processed all of this. After several minutes, I turned to him. "OK," I said. "Good," he replied, shoving me back down on the couch. "Then be a good boy, and keep your mouth shut until Daddy tells you to open it." He said those words, and something in my brain clicked. The endorphins started to rush, I felt flushed and tingly, and Daddy returned his attentions to my cock. He had found my breaking point and was careful to make sure that I didn't come. Over the next hour, he repeatedly brought me to the verge of orgasm, then backed down. After a few repetitions of this, I heard myself crying out, begging him to let me come, make me come. I've never begged anyone for anything, sex included, yet here I was, begging, whimpering, pleading with this man to bring me to orgasm. Through his actions, he staunchly refused. And I was loving it.

He stood up, and stared me up and down. He reached out both hands. I grabbed them, and he pulled me to a standing position, wrapping both arms around me, clutching me to his chest. I wobbled on legs that weren't yet fit to stand on.

"Can you stand up?" he whispered. "Ugghh . . ." I gurgled. "Good, then get down there like a good boy and help Daddy out of these clothes." he said, gently lowering me to the floor.

I untied his shoes and took off his socks. Looking up, I saw him looking down at me, beaming. I rose to my knees, and reached my hands up toward his belt. "That's it . . ." he cooed, running his hands through my hair, and resting them on my shoulders. I unbuckled his belt and unbuttoned his trousers. Stepping out of the pants, he stood there above me in plaid flannel boxers. I hesitated for a moment, then I pulled the shorts down, exposing his half-hard penis.

Nine inches indeed. It was huge, frighteningly so. I reached to grab it, and he grabbed me by the wrist. "No," he said. "Do you want to suck Daddy's cock?" I nodded, slightly. "Do you want to suck Daddy's cock?" he repeated. Again, I nodded, with a little more conviction this time. "Do? You? Want? To? Suck? Daddy's? Cock?" he asked, enunciating each word slowly and distinctly. "Yes, Daddy," I whispered, feeling very small and timid.

He grabbed his dick, held it right in front of my face, and slapped it against my cheek. Something I did must have told him I liked that, because he did it several more times, each time a little harder than the last. I could feel him getting harder with every slap. I opened my mouth to say something, and he stuffed his dick into my mouth. I gagged as the head of his cock hit the back of my throat. He grabbed me by the hair, and forced me to swallow more. "Relax," he said. "Daddy's a big boy. I'll teach you how to take it all. Just relax, breathe, and trust your daddy."

He pulled himself out, and lay down on the floor. I lay down next to him. He put his arm under my neck and with his other hand began stroking my cock. Slowly at first, but he worked his way up to a furious pace. I was writhing on the floor, panting, moaning, and begging Daddy to let me come. Again, he stopped just short of my orgasm. He slowed down for a few minutes, then speeded up again. "You want to come?" he asked, breathing heavily through gritted teeth. "Yes, please Daddy," I pleaded. He leaned over and licked my ear. "Then come for Daddy," he growled into my ear. And I did. I came with a scream. With enough force that a gob of semen landed with a wet smack on my Daddy's chin.

"That's my good boy . . ." I heard him say as I drifted off to sleep.

4.

I woke up maybe half an hour later.

Somehow, a pillow had ended up under my head, and a large blanket was covering me. I put on my boxers and followed the noises I heard to the kitchen. Philip stood at the stove, laboring over what looked like homemade spaghetti sauce. He turned and smiled at me. "I hope you're hungry," he said. We ate at the small table in his kitchen, mostly silently. "How was that?" he asked. "Amazing," I replied. I finished my pasta, and started to get up to put my plate in the sink. "No," Philip said, putting down his fork. He picked up my plate, took it to the sink, and sat back down across from me. He picked up his fork, and resumed eating. "Are you up for more?" he asked. "Would you like me to be?" I replied. "Yes." We spent the rest of that night playing together.

As things progressed, we both got more involved in our roles. He became aggressive, and I let go of more control. It was amazing. He was gentle and demanding, rough and sweet all at once. And not once did I feel unsafe. He was right, all I had to do was relax, and trust my daddy. He took care of me, and no matter what, put my pleasure ahead of his own.

We got together several more times after that first meeting. Sometimes, we'd just walk down to the diner on the corner and have omelets and pancakes for dinner. We'd talk about work and life, then we'd part ways with a friendly kiss on the cheek. Other times, we'd skip the meal all together and stay inside. Either way, he took care of me. I'd like to think I took care of him, too. I never expected that I would be able to get into the role-playing games we played, much less learn to enjoy it, relish it, but I began to look forward to the time we spent together. When I was with my daddy, all I wanted was to be a Good Boy.

Friends asked if he made me call him Daddy, and I explained that no one made me do anything. He was Daddy because I wanted him to be. The experience was not demeaning or demoralizing. Far from it. Philip taught me how good it feels to be taken care of, and that being powerful isn't always about being in control. This is a lesson I was glad to learn, something that I think will serve me well outside of the bedroom as well.

He also taught me a few other things, but those, dear reader, are another story.

The Cripple Liberation Front
Marching Band Blues
(Chapter 6)

Lorenzo W. Milam

I wish I could remember his name. I wish I had a clue. Maybe I would like to look him up, see what he looks like, now, at age thirty-nine. He probably has an admirable wife, two admirable children (fourteen and nine), and an admirable house with crushed stone on the driveway and gold lamé threads in the sofa, paintings by the Keenes on the walls. He probably can't even remember *my* name.

It is all just as well: that I have forgotten who he was, and all. He was the last of my child-innocent loves. For the life of me I can't remember if he is Frank or Tommy. Or Pat or Roger. So, I shall take the liberty of calling him a name of my own choosing: Randall, my son.

I wish I could tell you that my earliest love is beautiful, supple as the wind, body classically sculpted of Greek stone. I wish I could tell you that his muscles rippled beneath that marblelike exterior, that his eyes, a haunting blue-green, turned crystal sparkfire when the two of us were together. I would like to say that from his lips came the most arcane (and yet the most poetic) iambics of the land. I wish I could tell you all that.

Alas, it isn't so. As best I can remember, Randall's eyes are set too far apart: what would be called almond-eyes in others we will have to refer to as, uh, slightly piggy. His round fifteen-year-old face is nicely set off with a sprinkling of pimples. His mouth is far too wide and moist to be lovable to anyone. Except, possibly, his mother. And the long thin stranger in the next bed over, to the North.

Randall is fifteen years, three months old. He comes to Hopeless Haven in late November. He has diagnosed osteomyelitis. It is a cancerlike disease. The observation period is to see if the progress of the disease has been arrested, or whether it will continue to kill him.

To the few people who have known my love Randall, he is a typical middle South 1952 teenage boy with pimples and terminal shyness. Inside, he is replete with the vicious cells which sap the marrow of the bone, suck it dry, turn it to dust, visit death on the young and the innocent.

Inside Randall, as well, there is an affliction of supreme, radiant gentleness and a sly and quick humor. Just the thing that would appeal to his new next-door neighbor (some thirty inches away) at the particularly confused, anxious juncture of both of their lives.

Isn't that the way it works! Just when you have been visited by the gods who tell you that you don't have a chance, that all is lost, that you are nothing, that life is nothing, that there is no reason at all, at *all* for surviving, that you might as well hang it up, just hang it up: along comes some shy, bumbling, open-faced kid, just pops up like that right next to you and all of a sudden there is a softness and a light to all the white-and-shiny things which, days before, were so clinical and dull.

Walls take on a new hue. People seem kinder, or more human. Nurse Stumpf essays a smile for once in her dreadnought life. The sun peeps out from the thunderheads, and one night, at eleven or so, you can see a sliver of fall silver-powder moonlight that creeps along the ward floor. There is a gentleness in the air and a reason to wake up in the morning. The banging and caterwauling of the kids somehow seems less bruising, and you can lie with your love and be charged three thousand kilowatts with the sweet dew of kindness that turns your insides to bubbling gold.

There is a bizarre custom in that hopeless place: one that I recommend to all other hospitals, large and small. It is visitation. Not of the divine kind: those are reserved to the sallow-faced holies who plague our Sunday mornings with their chocolate-coated words. Nor am I speaking of the familial order—the ones who are allowed to materialize on Sunday afternoons from two to four.

No—I am speaking of visitations between patients, between the able-bodied and the disabled. In that stark setting, there is no place to sit. Certainly no isolated room with chairs. In a ward crowded with four dozen persons, no privacy is possible except under the scanty covers, and hardly there.

So when folks visit back and forth, they do so side by side, in the same bed. When Randall visits me, he lies on the bed next to me, his warm body threatening, by its very presence, to consume my own in a pure blue flame which seems to emanate, by magic, from his pores. He doesn't know his melting kindness, the effect it has on iceberg me. Or does he?

No questions asked. Visiting time is usually in the evening, before lights out. No suggestions of queer. A simple and a nice custom, for an otherwise gross environment.

I have no idea what we talk of, Randall and I. I don't know if we visit eighteen or twenty or three dozen times, or every day for three months. All I know is that in the midst of the arctic night of emotional despair, there is a glow. A candle, somewhere, is lit, briefly. Its flame gutters—then burns strongly, sending warm shadows through the otherwise dark room. There is given to us the knowledge that the two of us are neither totally nor irrecoverably alone.

For him and for me some bleak stranger has come down the road and pushed us off in the mud ditch. I, perhaps, shall never walk again. He may be dead within a year from the beast that eats away at his marrow. No matter: we have a respite from that. We are together. There is a chance that I have my arm under his neck. I am sure that from time to time I touch him with my hand. We may laugh together, leaning together in our quiet mirth, something for the two of us, something which, for a change, is ours alone, something that cannot be taken away from us by the rest of the maelstrom of the ward.

Randall and I. The two of us. The innocents in bed, in love to-gether. I can see the glint in his eyes as he whispers to me some partic-ular story out of his youth, or as he gives me a sly report on one of our wardmates. Our laughter is quiet, mixes quietly with the general bab-ble of the ward, and the ten radios competing with one another to be heard.

I can see him as he walks toward me across the ward. His hair hangs down across his forehead; he grins shyly. He walks, body turned slightly to the left, favoring the leg where the disease is eating the bone alive, the rich young marrow that feeds an insatiable disease.

It may have killed him, that disease, wasting him away. Or, as they operated on him again and again, trying to stop the inevitable "prog-ress" of the disease, his walk may have been turned to a crawling sluglike limp.

I don't want to think about that, and I shan't. Just as I have drawn a heavy black felt curtain, a curtain of mourning, over the fires of September, I shall draw a thick, humid, nightblue cloth over the two of us, Randall and I, at eight or eight-thirty of a dark November evening. We are carrying on about some unimportant, inconclusive bit of trivia; every now and then my hand touches his shoulder or arm, to emphasize a point, to let us know, us both know, that we are, after all, human, even though our bodies are their own friable element. There is in us some strong stuff of humanity: a warmth that fills us both, the cracked bowls replete with some sweet-smelling liquid.

I could, I suppose, go find him: somewhere, perhaps in northern Florida. He would be almost forty now. Or he would be dead. Either way, it would give me little. I loved him, deeply, when I did—and now I have covered him with a fine blue curtain.

Night Murmurs

John R. Killacky

I dissociate from the burning in my legs,
silently crying between sleep and the morning.
Hopes and dreams keep me safe through the night.

After surgery, I died then,
but you refused and brought me back.
Seven years and counting, of tilting toward the ground.

I'm afraid if I sit down; I'll never get up again.

Rehab gave me range of motion and strength.
Still, imaging a body I cannot have,
I want the cane to be temporary and no hand controls for the car.

Therapists caution about wear and tear,
while friends cheer, "You're getting better!"
I startle myself, glimpsing my fatigue in passing windows.

If I sit down, I'll never get up again.

Navigating my deadened limbs and twisted trunk,
pain remains constant, dulling our life together.
After a day's activities, I have no comfort left to give you.

When asked what you wanted, you hesitated, then said
"A wheelchair, so we could do more things together."
Only heroes aren't supposed to falter, aren't supposed to fail.

I'm afraid if I sit down, I'll never get up again.
If I sit down, I'll never get up again.

Beginner's Sex

Alex Sendham

My sex life was the pits until my accident.

True, there was my marriage and the children, and prodigious love lavished and lost (it seemed) by my mid-twenties, but pure rutting sexual congress hadn't made it to my right hemisphere yet. It was all beginner's sex.

I had other things to do. I wanted to make it as a sports pro and, equally, to make the Great American Documentary. And I was sure I could have the great American relationship later on when things were less hectic. I think it's called sublimation.

It took a spinal cord injury to wake me up. Even then, it wasn't cake. After I'd been lying around the hospital for a few days and was trying to make friends with the idea that ambulation/urination/defecation were going to be different, if not entirely absent, a doctor casually asked me if I was having erections. Erections? My god, it hadn't occurred to me. You have to be really perverse to ask a question like that at a time like this. It's like asking if I'm enjoying being paralyzed.

But doctors are perverse, and so is spinal cord injury, and this gig was turning out to be even more fun than I expected. Damn, I thought, he's probably going to tell me to forget about a climax, too. I was thirty-one years old.

(A decent period ensues to respect my privacy and battered ego. In my Great American Documentary, autumn leaves blow to a snowbound landscape. Presently, courageously, tentatively, the story resumes.)

There are rewards to being young enough to tempt and experienced enough to seduce. And, mark this, vulnerable. Sex and vulnerability go together like, well, like love and marriage. I wasn't out of the hospital a week before a student nurse from the psych shop next door, who also happened to live in the next apartment, popped in to chat. Cathy was determined to show me that I was still desirable, and she did a fine job of it. By the time she moved on to other peoples' vulnerabilities, she had pretty well convinced me that there is sex beyond erectile dysfunction.

But it took Sabrina to bring out the voluptuary in me. She had a manner I just couldn't stand and was pushy as hell about spending a lot of time at my place. I needed the latter, I guess, but I didn't enjoy her company all that much. Then truth revealed itself in the form of her multiple orgasms. It's a phenomenon I was coming to witness a little late in life, but Sabrina was a veritable gusher and I, as they say, ate it up.

"It gives you so much power over me," she said, and I was hooked. "I'm not sure I like that," she said. Doubly hooked. I hadn't understood that power and sex were connected. I hadn't understood that attraction and repulsion were two ends of the same stick, called sex.

We started exercising the power, once found, over each other. One night she would tell me what to wear for dinner—it might be my birthday suit or something outlandish like a coat and tie and jock strap—and the next night I would reciprocate, demanding clothing that was revealing, embarrassing, or somehow symbolic of sexual principles we never discussed but osmotically shared. She might make me put an ice cube in my shirt pocket until dinner was done, its steady cold drip making me hot, not cold. I would put Vaseline on her breasts so her T-shirt would stick to them, or paint animalistic designs on her thighs. Once she wanted to catheterize me, so she did.

It's manipulative and repellent to some, I suppose, but what we always did was whatever we thought would excite the other. That is, the person being told what to do was actually running the show because the other was trying to please. Neither of us ever learned whether we liked the telling or the being told better.

Sabrina would require me to wear something to work to act as a constant reminder—maybe a fetish to wear under clothing or a tie that had strong associations. Maybe an extra pair of shorts, or no shorts, to be silly. I would write limericks for her to wear in her panties, not to be read until work's end, or put a boiled egg in her pocket, a tangerine in her purse. For someone who has lost the explosive release of orgasm, a key concept is to prolong more sustainable levels of excitement. Don't think kettle drum, think slow brushes on the snares.

I tell you, it works. For the first time in my life, there was horniness all the live-long day and the promise of some fun at the end of it.

And what a high order of fun. Not everyone is turned on by oral sex, but if you are, you're automatically twice as interesting a partner as someone who isn't. That's for nondisabled people. For crips, it's orders of magnitude. It's the vehicle for both you and your mate to go as far as you want for as long as you want with no old-fashioned limitations such as premature ejaculation.

Add on the power trip, whatever you invent. Keep in mind that it's just reciprocal and consensual stuff between two adults who want to stay in each others' minds and pants all day long. Try it and then tell me it's sick.

It gets worse. See, Sabrina and I were having dessert one night— I think she had told me to dress up as a near-naked man with a baked potato in my jockeys, not too hot, no sour cream—when Old Nick whispered softly in my ear and said, "Take some of that warm chocolate syrup you're wasting on the vanilla ice cream and put it between those other lips."

I was entirely shocked by the idea, but that's what I did and that's when I learned that I love kinky sex. And had dessert.

And that, dear reader, is where I have to leave the subject because if you haven't thought of it yourself, or had your very own devil whisper sweet nothings in your ear, then the kink isn't real.

Sabrina and I lasted about two years. The sex never faded but the rest of our act did, thus proving the old saw that sex alone isn't enough. Well, it's not proof, yet in the fullness of my maturity its truth persists. We drifted apart, the sex lives on. No, that's wrong; it's the memory of it that lives on. I miss it. No, no, I definitely do not miss Sabrina. I thought we had already discussed that.

There were others. Beautiful blonde Joan—easy to live with, two adorable kids who got along well with my kids, she and I totally compatible. That's what killed that one. Marty, the speech pathologist, could not love me dear so much loved she not another more. Sarah, the filmmaker, dancer, poet, and novelist, was exactly the person I had looked for all my life, so naturally that didn't work out either. But life was full, sex was fulfilling.

And then, unaccountably, I turned gay.

It would trouble me if you thought that sex after paraplegia was so boring that the poor bugger—me, not to put too fine a point on it—

had to look around for novelty. What's next, you'll say. Sheep? Melons? You'll think that anyway, of course, because I've already told you I like kinky sex. Forget it. I was a late bloomer coming into sex at all, late into kink and really late into gay sex.

I'm not sure what precipitated the change. I'd always had a fascination with androgyny and same-sex love and, like most people who were sufficiently star-crossed to attend high school during the 1950s, I was scared to death of them. I've always been drawn to things that scare me.

My first experience of gay sex wasn't auspicious. It happened with someone I'd known for years, at a time when several other people I'd known for years, all straight, were crashing at my apartment. I'll spare you the fumbling details and just tell you that at evening's end my partner, using his midway barker's voice—for that's what he was—announced to all the friends in the next room who were rupturing their eardrums trying not to listen, "Sendham, you're the worst cocksucker I ever met."

I think he meant to spare my feelings.

Perhaps he meant to reassure the other guests in the apartment that we weren't either of us really gay. Maybe he was just stating a fact. In any case, he had the contrary effect of forcing me across the Rubicon. It was beginner's sex all over again.

It was surreal. In a lifetime of specializing in unintended seismic change, this was a tidal wave. It placed me squarely in a world that values youth and hard bodies even more than the dominant culture does, and I didn't know a soul who self-identified as gay.

It took a few years to find like-minded friends, and much longer to get comfortable in the cruising grounds of Queerlandia or feel liberated from the uncomfortable limbo—between the impulse and the deed, between women and men, between that kind of chum and this kind of chum—that I occupied like a spy behind enemy lines. It started with self-exploration and an assist from a surrogate sex partner that was readily available in nature.

It took me years to realize that I'd even missed it—the excitement of the wind riffling the hair on my body and creating that electric sense of nakedness and sexual acuity I'd feel when skiing fast or rock climbing on a windy day. Wearing shorts, of course, I could savor it in public, feel the breezes murmuring in the hair on my inner thighs. I'd skip the underwear to allow the free movement of air to stroke my imagination and sometimes my genitals. I'd climb trees naked, and sit high on a limb with my own limbs spread to life's own breath. Experienced apart from the realities of my sex life—defined as those parts I shared with others—these moments were the repeated reassurance that everything was possible, that all potential would be realized.

It's not the same from a wheelchair. In the presence of catheters and collection devices, who would expose himself at all? Why celebrate the inability to stand and feel where sensation had once been so keen? There's something erotically constipating about never getting air to your balls.

I lack sensation in my penis and testicles. Bad luck. But the hair—that's something different! A light silk scarf or a cashmere sweater drawn slowly, ever so slowly, over the genitals creates exquisite sensations. The bristly texture of a horsehair rope, moving millimeter by millimeter, makes me writhe and cry aloud. A light touch is an erotic promise made and delivered. A heavy touch is a clumsy confirmation of loss, no more, no less. The light touch is the lewd touch.

Rain. A leafy branch. Human breath.

But what is the softest, most capricious caress of all? The most intimate, yet most enveloping? The wind, of course. I am fortunate to live on a breezy hill affording total privacy, and I spent hours lying on a chaise with my thighs spread wide responding to the wind, to the atmosphere, to the stars. When I discovered stall bars—inexpensive homemade frames that allowed me to stand up unaided—I put them on three sides of the house so I could bare myself to the sun and wind coming from any quarter.

But the best and most satisfying tryst with the wind came one night in the back of Tyler's pickup. I threw a pad from that same chaise into the truck's bed, stripped, then transferred onto the pad face up. I wanted to be helpless, so Tyler tied my arms and legs to the four corners of the truck bed. He added another touch; he painted strong Mentholatum on my nipples, and then did it again. It hurt, but it was a hurt that felt lascivious and good.

Did I tell you? It was a windy Halloween kind of night, and when the truck drove off my excitement was nearly unbearable. Fingers of wind licked at every pore of my body, made every nerve ending *feel* for the first time since my injury. My nipples were on fire from the Mentholatum—two fine, fiery points of light burning on my chest—

yet the stuff was also evaporating in the wind, a hot and cold contradiction that made me feel like my lungs were empty spaces and I had holes in my trunk like a Henry Moore sculpture. There was wind rushing through the holes and it was glorious.

As the pickup reached cruising speed, the fingers of wind started kneading and coaxing, exploring and penetrating and fucking and sucking and driving my body and I started to sing, I thought, but the song became a sustained moan—an emanation, really—that I could no more control than I had once been able to control the last stages of an orgasm. It was coming from my entire body and it kept coming until something in it was satisfied. There were radiating currents of electricity and fire and thrilling cold, and their expression was holy sound.

We turned into the long driveway that leads to Tyler's house, and bounced slowly along the cattle track that serves as a roadbed. A mile of humping through ruts and creek beds and over cattle guards gave me barely enough time to silence the song of the wind.

I didn't have to explain to Tyler how it had been. He knew. I don't know how, but he knew.

"That was wonderful," he said.

Tyler has a house in Montana where he and I spent one moonlit evening drinking and alternating between whatever we could think of to do sexually and relaxing in the sauna. It's a nice combination and we were both feeling pretty good already, but of course we wanted to do something more, always more.

There's a beaver pond right in front of the house filled with the coldest water on earth. It has a dock I can wheel out on, so I hooked the kayak's grab loop over one of the push handles of my wheelchair, dragged it onto the dock, and made the dicey transfer to the boat. Naked, of course, and I didn't wear a spray skirt to keep the water out of the cockpit—I wanted to feel it all. Kayak and I ottered into the water.

It was one of the most crystalline and sensual experiences of my life. My body carried all that heat from the sauna, so the cold air and water were only added stimulants. I paddled with a child's fresh sense of play, the kayak's bow knifing, carving and surfing, a thousand reflected moons sucked down into the eddies and swirls I was creating with each stroke. Drops of water on the paddle blade caught the moonlight like diamonds, then fell on my thighs and belly and cock and balls like sparks from a welding rod, and there was something in that cadenced rain of icy fire that creates in me yet a memory of unblemished innocence and well-being.

But have there been people? you might ask. The kink is one thing, I'm sure you think, but where's the beef? Excuse me, but where are the solid family values we all know to be the root of earthly happiness? Where are the other dimensions of relationship and sexuality?

I'll tell you about some of it. My ex-wife and I have, over forty-one years, jointly raised our children and shared the praise and blame. We meet often and get along well; she's happily married, I'm happily divorced, and the marriage and its issue are still sacred commitments in my life. In a sense, it has turned into the great American relationship I once deferred, just more extended than I anticipated. Her husband is a well-loved member of our family, as is Tyler, and both visit frequently. The kids have turned out exceedingly well, the grandkids have been arriving now for years, and our lives are all very much intertwined. It seems like a tight family. Everyone knows I'm gay and everyone tolerates it. That's four generations of support, including my parents but not the dog.

And is there still sex after all these years? Not so much, but I like being an old fart. One could do worse. Maybe I'll get laid when I'm not so busy. Or maybe I'll just slide out slow and easy, with enough sex behind me, nothing missed and no regrets.

Queer Ducks: An Unlikely Romance

Donald H. Lawrence Jr.

Did I say "unlikely"? You be the judge. I was born in 1947 in Brooklyn, New York; he was born in 1961 in Albuquerque, New Mexico. While he was growing up, getting a BFA in acting, marrying, parenting, and dancing flamenco, I was coming out after high school, dropping out of college in my first year, and actively alcoholic through the 1970s. Then, not too long ago, I retired (early) to North Carolina. Oh, and I'd sooner croak than be on a stage.

And if that's not enough, consider these facts as the basis for a romance: primary progressive multiple sclerosis (his) and limb-girdle muscular dystrophy and a ten-year-old colostomy (mine). The thing is, romance was not on the agenda. We met at my infant Web site for gay men with disabilities. I had not designed it as a lonely hearts club. Really.

It took two months for somebody—anybody—to find my site. The somebody was Bruce. We were the only members . . . until it was too late.

He introduced himself as Scotch-Irish (heavy on the Scotch) and a former flamenco dancer, thirty-eight-years-old, bisexual, with a "wonderful wife and two beautiful sons." So I'm thinking, nice. We don't have much in common, but I'm glad for another group member. I had lost my lover of eighteen years to cancer less than a year earlier, and I wasn't really thinking of romance. If I had been, my requisites would have been more like "fifty to sixty years or older, *homo*sexual, and, of course, SINGLE." I mean, shit, I saw all three versions of *Back Street,* so I just knew what I needed, if I needed anybody: someone nice and dull, plain and simple—not a friggin' flamenco dancer!

The thing was, through lots of e-mail, an undeniable chemistry was developing. I knew I was looking forward to Bruce's postings—much too much, in fact. Neither of us had any idea what the other looked like, though I did let Bruce know, early in our correspondence—way before the romantic detour—that I am black. Often,

199

people assume I'm something other, even in person, and I'm exposed to comments and thinking about black folks that I might be spared, if my race were more obvious, in the same way that you have probably been treated to fag jokes when your sexuality was unknown to the speaker. So, to preclude the need for activism in response, I try to make things clear in advance.

What I've found throughout my life is that people relate more on the basis of background and common experience than they do on the basis of race. I don't have everything in common with every black person. I have had a great deal in common with some people who aren't black. I found that Bruce and I shared values, interests, humor, music, movies, idiosyncrasies, sensitivities, sensibilities, politics. Our fourteen-year age difference made this more surprising than did our different races. Bruce's mother and father bore striking similarities to mine (his dad, my father, and I even share first and middle names: Donald Herbert). Our respective relationships with each of them were formative and almost identical.

Bruce has brothers near my age. He has absorbed their interests and experiences and culture, so our frames of reference are closer than one might expect. We discovered all of these things during months of e-mailing. Here and there, an oddly romantic note crept in. First, Bruce offered his personal e-mail address, so that we could by-pass my Web site. Then he commented that, ". . . this is like *You've Got Mail.*" Whoa, I thought . . . isn't that a ROmance?!

Then, he and the family went away for a weekend. We were both sort of dreading the separation. On their return, we had to admit we had missed each other "inordinately," a pet word for both of us. Maybe most significantly, there was the time I, emotionally, shared how much the death of my lover had impacted my life. Bruce e-mailed back: "Sir, if ever I might ease your pain." Gulpppp! I was a goner!

As we both admitted how important those e-mails had become, as we realized how our relationship was . . . shifting, we agreed on one thing above all else: we didn't want anything to interfere with Bruce's family or his place in it. There couldn't be any happiness for us if that were to happen, so I had no intention of calling Bruce's house, ever.

Bruce describes himself as a "compulsive confessor." It sounded to me like a rare kind of openness and honesty and it made his wife, Mary, privy to our correspondence from the start. Mary initiated an exchange with me that became a correspondence not only comfortable but at times quite independent of anything to do with Bruce. Mary had always known that Bruce wasn't "straight." They'd had, and have, a wonderful partnership, but she knew that there had been some sexual incompatibility, and she felt that this was a good opportunity for change. She encouraged us. More than that, she urged Bruce to "just come out," offering to "hold open the closet door" for him.

Was I surprised? Surprised?! I couldn't believe this was happening, or that I was going along with it. But I began to feel that having all of this develop, gradually, in spite of ourselves, was preordained. The universe was moving us together, wasn't it? We just had to get out of the way. This confidence in the inevitable overrode my instincts, which had been telling me to run for the hills.

And so, last Thanksgiving, I somehow got up the courage to go to Albuquerque to meet Bruce and Family in person. After the meeting at the airport, we picked up my rental car. Mary and the boys (Alex and Drew) helped Bruce into my car, put his wheelchair into my trunk and led us back home in their car. They put us alone, together, for the first time, after months and months of imagining it. Well, not exactly A-lone, but there in the car we could hold hands at last.

Back home, I was in for a real surprise. Mary ended all my logistical concerns about sleeping arrangements. She shot Bruce up with his double-blind experimental drug, and packed him off to stay the night with me at the motel. Are you amazed? As amazed as I was? I can't begin to describe my gratitude and happiness. But wait. She joined us at our room in the morning for the complimentary calorie blast.

I also can't describe how normal and comfortable this seemed. (Mary, when you read this, I LOVE YOU!) In a glorious week of acceptance, of hanging out with the family, another event stands out. Bruce and I had the pleasure of picking the boys up after school. One day, we were retrieving Alex from after-school care early, and he had to be signed for. When we pulled into the schoolyard, he came running over. I said I'd wait in the car while he and Bruce went in to sign out. "No, Don," Alex insisted, "you hafta come in and meet everybody!" This was waaaay beyond the call of duty. I knew then that he wasn't having a problem with us.

In March, Bruce came here to North Carolina for two weeks. On August twenty-third he returned for good, with lots of room to continue as part of his incredible family, through mutual visits. I'm a little defensive talking about the family issue, because I'd have never chosen to fall in love with a married man. Remember, I was born in 1947. It might as well have been the Victorian Era. I mean, we had . . . standards! But it was the family, Bruce's incredible, one-in-a-million family, which made it OK for me. Alex, eleven, met me at the airport that first time, holding a big "Don" sign he'd made. Drew, fifteen, gave his Dad a "Queer Duck" sweatshirt for Christmas, saying, "It's OK, Dad. I know you like ducks!" How do people get to be this remarkable? I wish I knew.

Our disabilities sometimes create physical challenges, but they make for a level of understanding and ease that I can't otherwise explain. How do you manage with dual disabilities? Maybe it's a matter of Faith versus Risk and Karma. The potentially scary part of a dual-disability relationship involves the unknown and unknowable progression of disease and incapacity that we each face.

At present, things work just fine. Bruce has more compromised mobility than I, but for now, at least, I am able to compensate. I have some compromised sexual function, but with Bruce's patience and tenacity (and humpiness), that is manageable and even improving. Horizontally, we are all but indistinguishable from any two lovers, except, maybe, that we are obsessive snuggle-cuddlers. One advantage conferred by the fact that we're both disabled is that we discussed all of our physical problems long before romance reared its head. We didn't face questions of "when," "how much," or "how soon" to disclose potentially troubling details. For example, since we've each had experience with messy incontinence issues, and will again, it's not the embarrassment it might be. Right now, we are relishing the present, the very unexpected chance for happiness that Providence has dished out.

Ever since I was a twink I have always thought of myself as practicing "sexual karma." The idea is simple: never say no. I fear rejection so much that I don't make advances. I figured if I didn't reject anyone else, even if I weren't particularly interested, that I might be rewarded with attention from some extraordinary people along the way, people I'd never have imagined for myself.

It's been the case. Bruce is proof absolute.

My advice, to contradict a former First Lady: "Just say yes!"

Bruce is, as usual, stretched out beside me as I write this. One advantage of disability is that no one expects us to be out plowing the south forty. My schnauzer is lying across Bruce's stomach, insisting on continuous petting. One cat is stopping the circulation in my legs and another is curled up at our feet. This leaves a Pomeranian and a third cat unaccounted for. They hang out together. We think they suffer from species-identity confusion disorder. They seem to be dealing with their confusion just fine.

As for us, well, we're not confused at all anymore.

It's All in the Eye: A Deaf Gay Man Remembers His Icons

Raymond Luczak

I left my hometown, Ironwood, Michigan, a good many years ago. The town I remember did not seem to have shrunk from the emptied iron-ore mines nearby, nor did it seem to thrive on the flocks of skiers and tourists that came through to look at Copper Peak, the largest ski jump in the Western Hemisphere, or Hiawatha, the world's tallest fiberglass statue. Ironwood seemed never to change, in spite of the decisive seasons we endured.

I was the one who changed; I was always different. I didn't know how to explain why, but I knew it involved far more than the hearing-aid harness I wore under my shirt like a bra. I was ashamed—although I hadn't quite grasped why at the time—to be deaf and to have imperfect and nasal speech. Moreover, I was skinny and non-athletic. When I matured a little more quickly than others, I found myself falling in love with my male classmates and teachers. Endlessly fascinated with them, I hadn't yet realized the sexual possibilities of connecting.

Just as my imperfect ears are able to grasp the bare skeletons of sound, I did not realize I was gay—or even identify with certain icons revered by gay men—in an instant Hollywood moment; it was more an epic journey than anything else. A cast of dozens, some of whose names I have forgotten, held up signposts that gleamed in the darkness of my wondering. I was constantly amazed that no one had ever caught them the way I had.

Because I live vicariously through my eyes, I am incapable of tossing snappy comebacks learned from the movies or mimicking lyrics from Broadway musicals. My memories of growing up gay are sealed tight in the Pandora's box of my eyes. I am always looking back to see where I've been and how far I've gone.

Out in the schoolyard, my best friend and I are fighting over the TV show *Batman*. The year is 1975; we are ten-year-old fourth graders. He is hearing, and he is my best friend because he doesn't care that I'm deaf, or that I have to spend half-days with his hearing class and half-days in my own deaf classroom. He says that Batman fights better than Robin. I disagree. We squabble over this nearly every day. I cannot help staring at Batman's firm jaw and the faint smile wrinkles underneath his mask, but I instinctively know it is not a thing to share. I finally give up watching the reruns after school, but the images of BRAAAAAAK! WHAM! never leave me.

Years later, after we'd moved apart, we connect and find that although he's been married for a long time, he's become bisexual. He acknowledges that he was in love with me then. Apparently we'd both recognized the same confused, subliminally campy signals that *Batman* had broadcast.

At fifteen, I am obsessed with Harrison Ford. His stubble in *Raiders of the Lost Ark* excites me, although in my dreams I am afraid to touch his jaw. He is clearly a man's man; why should he have anything to do with me? I'd been snubbed by hearing classmates only half as self-assured as Indiana Jones. The scene that replays itself most often in my mind involves Ford, his arm bandaged, lying in bed on a ship. Karen Allen, the hard-boiled heartthrob, bends over and kisses him. The scene plays out something like this: "It hurts here" (he says). She kisses where it hurts, then finally kisses him on the lips, where, Indy admits, it also hurts. It was the first time in the movies I felt the healing possibilities of a kiss.

I am seventeen years old and it is the night of the much-ballyhooed final episode of *M*A*S*H*. Everyone is packed into the living room, eyes glued to the screen. I sit upstairs, my eyes glued to a public library copy of Gerold Frank's *Judy,* perhaps the definitive biography of this century's greatest gay icon. Nowhere does it say anything about gay men, but the way Frank tells her story moves me to tears. In the background I hear claps and sobs and laughs from the TV watchers, but I don't care.

Judy and I are alone together, warm against the wintry world. I sigh over the passionate—and shamelessly horrendous—poems I write about her. There is something about her eyes, the way they travel from one person to another, as if in a dream. I imagine myself as Judy, and mouth the words to "Over the Rainbow" in front of the mirror. No sound comes out, for I know I cannot sing. I dream of seeing *A Star Is Born* after reading anecdote after anecdote about how difficult it was to make that film, and how triumphant a comeback it was for her. Years later, when I get my own closed-caption decoder for my TV and VCR, I discover that the movie isn't even captioned. I stare at the stills instead and imagine Judy as Esther, rising to the unimaginable top with her heart torn over her fallen star. It is my story, I imagine, where no one ever gets all of what they want.

My speech therapist at Bay Cliff Health Camp unnerves me. For one thing, my therapists had always been women. He is blond and slender like me; his glasses are thick but completely clear, without distortion. When he touches my throat as I try to perfect the more difficult dipthongs, I shrink away. I do not feel comfortable, or is it that his tastes—casually displayed in the cassette tapes of Mike Oldfield and Bruce Springsteen's early albums—are foreign to anything I've seen in Ironwood? I look at Springsteen smiling and gazing off into the distance, and I keep remembering his smile—it's as if he has something to hide. I look at my speech therapist and wonder whether *he* has any secrets, whether these albums were meant to hide secrets or reveal them.

My sister Jean brings home Elton John's *Rock of the Westies* album. I don't care for him, but I am fascinated by his smile and his stubble. Jean grooves to the album, while I cannot tear my eyes off Elton's. I look for his records in stores, and I wonder how he can get away with such flamboyant goofiness when I am such a total misfit in school, where I am not even allowed to wear slogans and funny pins. I wish more than ever that I could play the piano and sing. Years later, when I catch the last of Stockard Channing's performances in John Guare's *Six Degrees of Separation* at Lincoln Center, Elton John himself sits across the aisle, two rows back. I do not recognize him at first, but his intense gaze back at me frightens. What did I have to say to him? That the beard he sported in the 1970s would still look good on him? No.

The summer of 1979: I am in Ronnie's, Ironwood's premier record shop. I am completely taken with the album cover of the Village People's *Go West*. They are so handsome, so . . . confident. I wonder if any of them endured the agony of adolescent pimples. I buy "Macho Man," and I play the single over and over. Oh, did I want to be a macho man! But no one was willing to show me how. It seemed that everyone had the secret but me. Even then I cannot decode the fact that they are a bunch of gay men; my eyes roam the blatant hirsuteness of Glenn Hughes, the leatherman. When I look at the Village People posters his eyes never leave mine, but my fantasies are still innocent, not yet awakened in vividly sexual flavors.

The first time I saw Boy George on the cover of Culture Club's debut album, *Kissing to Be Clever,* I didn't know who that petulant girl was. A few weeks later, when I saw "Do You Really Want to Hurt Me?" on MTV, I realized she was much too tall to be a girl, and my sister said, "That's Boy George."

I bought the album anyway. He wasn't attractive to me, but the more I read about him, the more I secretly admired his outrageousness. My mother was horrified at the flashy green dress he donned for the 1983 Grammy Awards. I wanted to be as steely-eyed and nervy as he when he accepted the Grammy for Best New Artist with his unforgettable line, "Thank you, America, for recognizing a good drag queen when you see one." I nearly cried. Why should I be happy for a triumphant drag queen? It wasn't as if I wanted to wear a dress myself.

I remember when I was ten, and seeing Bette Davis for the first time (with no idea who she was) in the Disney film *Return from Witch Mountain.* I don't remember much about the story, which was most likely negligible, but I do remember her eyes cutting a swath through whatever else was happening on the screen. Years later my hearing lover discovered that I'd never seen Joseph Mankiewicz's *All About Eve.* He was infuriated to find that the videotape was not closed-captioned. "How can deaf gay people understand the hearing gay community if they can't understand their movies?" By chance, he found a jacket-less hardback of Gary Carey's *More About All About Eve* for ninety-nine cents in a Barnes & Noble cutout bin. Overjoyed, I read the script. I was struck by the acid banter and the suave insider-ness of the theater world (by that time I'd been writing plays myself), and then we watched Margo Channing have a go at the ambitious Eve Harrington. Although the script was fresh in my mind, I found myself at a loss. The truth of the story was not about the action on the screen; it was about action in the *voice,* in the voiceovers, in the mind. What could a deaf gay man glean from watching this movie? I could never hope to replicate its dialogue in American Sign Language, with its syntax and grammar completely different from English.

Such talky films remind me yet again how culturally different deaf gay men are from hearing gay men. We both love movies, but deaf gay viewers need the dialogue made accessible to them. It is not surprising, then, that the deaf gay community does not derive its cultural identity from movies (the majority of which are heterosexual and offer no subliminal homosexual context) or musicals (few of which are sign-interpreted) to the degree that hearing gay men do.

The day I saw the silver-sheen cover of Queen's album, *The Game,* which included their smash hits "Crazy Little Thing Called Love," and "Another One Bites the Dust," something inside my head went off. I couldn't figure out until years later that the vacant looks of Freddie Mercury and his band were identical to those of men in bars who didn't want to give too much of themselves away while waiting to be approached. And, of course, I was totally blind to the tongue-in-cheek irony of the group's name.

After I came out in 1984, as a college freshman, I paid more attention to a host of so-called gay icons, women such as Crawford, Dietrich, and Stanwyck, who displayed pathos, bitchiness, sassiness, vulnerability, and sexiness on the screen in ways that no man could match. As my insight expanded, I realized there could be no movie frame of reference common to both deaf gay and hearing gay men until films such as *Caged* and *All About Eve* are made accessible to the deaf.

It is clear that my icons were not necessarily traditionally gay in the pre-Stonewall sense; the books available at my hometown's public library, the few movies shown in town, and the types of records that were stocked and sold there, all combined with the silence on homosexuality, forced me to invent my own icons, even forced me to put words in their mouths. My experience reminds me of a deaf lesbian who had watched *The Wizard of Oz* a dozen times. When that film was closed-captioned at last, she was ecstatic, but then she discovered that no one said anything near what she'd imagined they'd been saying all along. Though she remained a Judy Garland fan, she was deeply disappointed.

Everywhere I went, my eyes photographed the sparks of glamour I was able to glean from all those icons. I remain a walking gallery of the images that brought me closer to the cliff, to the once-unknown place where I could at last come out as a deaf gay man. The images I captured with my eyes are part of my continuing plunge into the joyful chasm of being out, proof that my ears didn't have to make me alone.

Gawking, Gaping, Staring

Eli Clare

Gawking, gaping, staring: I can't say when it first happened. When first a pair of eyes caught me, held me in their vice grip, tore skin from muscle, muscle from bone. Those eyes always shouted, "Freak, retard, cripple," demanding an answer for tremoring hands, a tomboy's bold and unsteady gait I never grew out of. It started young, anywhere I encountered humans. Gawking, gaping, staring seeped into my bones, became the marrow. I spent thirty years shutting it out, slamming the door.

The gawkers never get it right, but what I want to know is this: will you? When my smile finds you across the room, will you notice the odd angle of my wrists cocked and decide I am a pane of glass to glance right through? Or will you smile back?

Thirty years, and now I am looking for lovers and teachers who will hold all my complexities and contradictions gently, honestly, appreciatively. Looking for heroes and role models who will accompany me through the world. Looking for friends and allies who will counter the gawking, gaping, staring.

I come from peoples who have long histories of being on stage— freaks and drag queens, court jesters and scientific experiments. Sometimes we work for money and are proud. Other times we're just desperate. We've posed for anthropologists and cringed in front of doctors, jumped through hoops and answered the same questions over and over, performed the greatest spectacles and thumbed our noses at that shadow they call normal.

William Johnson—African American and cognitively disabled in the mid-1800s—worked the freak-show stage. He donned an ape costume and shaved his head, save for a tuft of hair at the very top, and became the monkey man, the missing link, the bridge between "brute" and "man." P. T. Barnum, showman extraordinaire and shaper of the institution of the freak show, named William's exhibit "What-Is-It?" People paid to gawk, and William died a well-off man. The folks who performed alongside William affectionately called him the "dean of freaks." Today that question—what is it?—still lingers, still haunts us, only now the gawkers get in for free.

Billy Tipton worked the jazz stage with his piano, saxophone, and comedy routines. Billy lived for fifty years as a female-bodied man. He married five times and adopted three sons. He turned down major, high-profile music gigs. He died of a bleeding ulcer rather than seeking out medical care. He was much admired by the men he played music with. This we know about Billy, but there is also much we don't know: how he thought of himself, his gender; what prompted him to make the move from woman to man; what went through his head as he lay dying in his son's arms. But really, the questions I want to ask aren't about his gender but rather about his life as a musician. *Billy, what did your body feel like as your fingers raced into a familiar song, playing in front of great throngs of people?* The gawking started after his death as the headlines roared, "Jazz Musician Spent Life Concealing Fantastic Secret."

I listen to the histories and everywhere hear the words *cripple, queer, gimp, freak:* those words hurled at me, those words used with pride. When I walk through the world, the bashers see a fag, the dykes see a butch, and I myself don't have many words. I often leave it at genderqueer or transgender butch. The gawkers never get it right. They think I'm deaf or "mentally retarded." They think I'm a twenty-one-year-old guy or a middle-aged dyke. They can't make up their minds, start with sir, end with ma'am, waver in the middle. They think I am that pane of glass.

Cripples, queers, gimps, freaks: we are looking for lovers and teachers—teachers to stand with us against the gawking; lovers to reach beneath our clothing, beneath the words that attempt to name us, beneath our shame and armor, their eyes and hands helping return us to grace, beauty, passion. *He cradles my right hand against his body and says, "Your tremors feel so good." And says, "I can't get enough of your shaky touch." And says, "I love your cerebral palsy." This man who is my lover. Shame and disbelief flood my body, drowning his words. How do I begin to learn his lustful gaze?*

Believing him takes more than trust. I spent so many years shutting the staring out, slamming the door. Friends would ask, "Did you see that person gaping at you?" and I'd answer, "What person?" It's a great survival strategy but not very selective. In truth the door slammed hard, and I lost it all, all the appreciation, flirtation, solidarity that can be wrapped into a gaze. These days I practice gawking at the gawkers and flirting as hard as I know how. The first is an act of resistance; the second, an act of pride. I am looking for teachers.

If I had a time machine, I'd travel back to the freak show. Sneak in after hours, after all the folks who worked long days selling themselves as armless wonders and wild savages had stepped off their platforms, out of their geek pits, from behind their curtains. I'd walk among them—the fat women, the short-statured men commonly called dwarves and midgets, the folks without legs, the supposed half-men/half-women, the conjoined twins, the bearded women, the snake charmers and sword swallowers—as they took off their costumes, washed their faces, sat down to dinner. I'd gather their words, their laughter, their scorn at the customers—the rubes—who bought their trinkets and believed half their lies. I'd breathe their fierceness into me.

I am looking for teachers and heroes to show me the way toward new pride, new understanding, new strength, a bigger sense of self. Often it is history I turn to, history I grasp and mold in my search. I am not alone in this endeavor. I think of a kid we've come to know as Brandon Teena: twenty-one years old, living as a guy in rural Nebraska, revealed as female-bodied, raped, and murdered by so-called friends. In trans community, we've chosen him. Claimed him as an FTM (a female-to-male trans person) based on how his life makes sense to us without listening to his confusion. Named him Brandon Teena without paying attention to the dozen other names he used. We have made him hero, martyr, symbol of transphobic violence. I think again of Billy Tipton. In the lesbian community, many have taken Billy to be an emblem of the sexism in the jazz world of the mid-1900s. They shape his life as a man into a simple survival strategy that allowed him to play music. I myself read the life of William Johnson and find someone who turned a set of oppressive material and social conditions to his benefit and gained a measure of success and community. That reading strengthens me. But in truth William might have been a lonely, frightened man, coerced, bullied, trapped by freak-show owners and managers. We use and reshape history, and in the process it sometimes gets misshapen.

At the same time, we all need teachers and heroes: folks to say, "You're not alone. I too was here. This is what I did and what I learned. Maybe it'll help." My best heroes and teachers don't live on pedestals. They lead complex, messy lives, offering me reflections of myself and standing with me against the gawkers.

The gawkers who never get it right. They've turned away from me, laughed, thrown rocks, pointed their fingers, quoted Bible verses, called me immoral and depraved, tried to heal me, swamped me in pity. Their hatred snarls into me, and often I can't separate the homophobia from the ableism from the transphobia.

The gawkers never get it right, but what I want to know is this: will you? If I touch you with tremoring hands, will you wince away, thinking cripple, *thinking* ugly*? Or will you unfold to my body, let my trembling shimmer beneath your skin?*

These days, I practice overt resistance and unabashed pride, gawking at the gawkers and flirting as hard as I know how. The two go together. On the Castro, I check out the bears, those big burly men with full beards and open shirts. One of them catches my eyes. I hold his gaze for a single moment too long, watch as it slips down my body. He asks, "Are you a boy or a girl?" not taunting but curious. I don't answer. What could I possibly say? I walk away smiling, my skin warm.

In another world at another time, I would have grown up neither boy nor girl, but something entirely different. In English there are no good words, no easy words. All the language we have created—transgender, transsexual, drag queen, drag king, stone butch, high femme, nellie, fairy, bulldyke, he-she, FTM, MTF (a male-to-female trans person)—places us in relationship to masculine or feminine, between the two, combining the two, moving from one to the other. I'm hungry for an image to describe my gendered self, something more than the shadowland of neither man nor woman, more than a suspension bridge tethered between negatives. I want a solid ground with bedrock of its own, a language to take me to a brand new place neither masculine nor feminine, day nor night, mortise nor tenon. What could I possibly say to the bears cruising me at 3 p.m. as sunlight streams over concrete?

Without language to name myself, I am in particular need of role models. I think many of us are. Who do we shape our masculinities, our femininities, after? Who shows us how to be a drag queen, a butch, a trannyfag (a gay FTM) who used to be a straight married woman and now cruises the boys hot and heavy, a multigendered femme boy/girl who walks the dividing line? I keep looking for disabled men to nurture my queer masculinity, crip style. Looking for bodies a bit off-center, a bit off-balance. Looking for guys who walk with a tremble; speak with a slur; who use wheelchairs, crutches, ventilators, braces; whose disabilities shape, but don't contradict, their masculinities.

And in truth I am finding those role models. There is a freak show photo: Hiram and Barney Davis offstage—small, wiry men, white, cognitively disabled, raised in Ohio. They wear goatees, hair falling past their shoulders. They look mildly and directly into the camera. Onstage, Hiram and Barney played "Waino and Plutano, the Wild Men of Borneo." They snapped, snarled, growled, shook their chains at the audience. People flocked to the "Wild Men," handing over good money to gape. I hope just once Hiram and Barney stopped mid-performance, up there on the sideshow platform, and stared back, turning their mild and direct gaze to the rubes, gawking at the gawkers.

It usually takes only one long glance at the gawkers—kids on their way home from school, old women with their grocery bags, young professionals dressed for work. Just once I want someone to tell me what they're staring at. My tremoring hands? My buzzed hair? My broad, off-center stance, shoulders well-muscled and lopsided? My slurred speech? Just once. But typically one long, steely glance, and they're gone. I am taking Hiram and Barney as my teachers.

The gawkers never get it right, and what I want to know is this: will you? When I walk through the world, will you simply scramble for the correct pronoun, failing whichever one you choose, he not all the way right, she not all the way wrong? Or will you imagine a river at dusk, its skin smooth and unbroken, sun no longer braided into sparkles? Cliff divers hurl their bodies from thirty, forty, fifty feet, bodies neither flying nor earth-bound, three somersaults and a half turn, entering the water free-fall without a ripple. Will you get it right?

I am looking for friends and allies, for communities where the staring, gaping, gawking finally turns to something else, something true to the bone. Places where strength gets to be softened and tempered, love honed and stretched. Where gender is known as more than a simple binary. Where we are encouraged to swish and swagger, limp and roll, and learn the language of pride. Places where our bodies begin to become home. Gawking, gaping, staring: I can't say when it first happened.

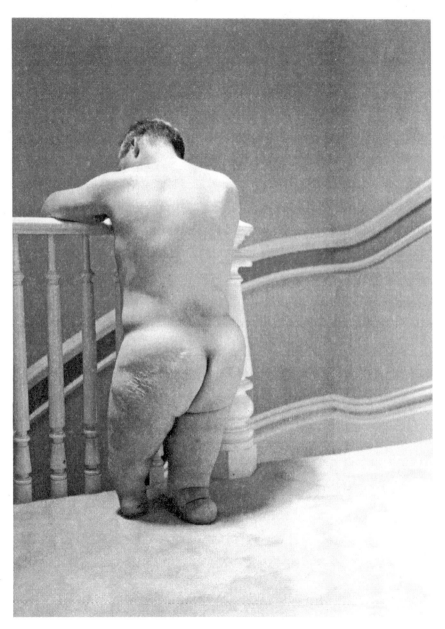

Destination *Bent:*
The Story Behind a Cyber Community
for Gay Men with Disabilities

Bob Guter

To this day I cannot stomach the taste of orange sherbet. When I was a very small child, orange sherbet was the favored hospital treat, used to calm anesthesia-heaved innards and distract small patients from the sudden disappearance of visiting parents. I spent a lot of time in a lot of hospitals when I was a very small child.

> This child has a congenital absence of all fingers on the right hand and a rudimentary thumb. The cause of these deformities is unknown. The thumb is loosely articulated with the lower end of the radius. The rudimentary right hand exhibits some active flexion of the soft carpal mass but no voluntary action of the thumb. Whether or not this flexor action can be utilized for activating a prosthesis is questionable. This child also exhibits a congenitally dislocated hip and deformities of both lower legs with congenital absence of fibula. There is a severe bowing deformity with associated *equinus* deformity of both feet. With respect to the congenital deformity of both lower extremities, I strongly recommend amputation of both feet by disarticulation, leaving below-the-knee stumps.

So wrote Henry H. Kessler, renowned surgeon, rehabilitation pioneer, founder of the Kessler Institute for Rehabilitation. "This child" was me, at the age of five.

My father's horrified reaction was to spend the next year searching for "better" advice. After being told repeatedly, "Kessler knows best," he took me back to the Great Man, who brushed off my father's apologies and proceeded with the disarticulation he had recommended a year before. I know these details only because my father recited them to me in one of a series of conversations we had the year before he died. I think of those talks and similar halting conversations throughout the years as family archaeology, a belated attempt to piece together our own lost civilization. We dug up shards, brushed off the dirt, analyzed, catalogued: I learned that I was not shown to my mother for a week after birth; that she then had a nervous breakdown. I learned that she blamed my father for what "happened," and that he blamed her.

I learned that before Dr. Kessler's evaluation, I had undergone corrective surgeries by several different surgeons in several different hospitals. None of the surgeries corrected anything. Decades later, when I ask my mother exactly how many operations, how many hospitals, she cannot . . . remember.

It's not only my mother who cannot remember. Except for a few scraps, most everything about the physical details of what it was like to be me before the age of six are lost. All those preamputation years—when I crawled or was carried but never walked—are vaporized. I do remember repeated ether dreams, almost impossible to describe if you haven't had one. And with special vividness I remember one occasion when my father held me in his arms in a hospital corridor somewhere, with a view down into a courtyard five or six floors below. Someone approached with food on a tray. I recall the *feeling* of being so angry (at what?) that I want to hurl the tray through the window and down into the courtyard. Rage, but impotent rage.

During one of my several adult tries at sorting things out through talk therapy, my therapist observed, "You have been suffering from post-traumatic stress disorder since you were born. Your parents, too. Today, of course, there's immediate and long-term therapy for everybody concerned in situations like yours, support groups, counseling at school . . ."

But coexistent with the blankness where I seem to have no physical existence, was an eminently physical feeling-state full of pleasurable longing. I remember wanting to hug and kiss older boys, always wanting to sit on the lap of my favorite handsome uncle and be petted by him. I remember my father's best friend and how his blond hairiness fascinated me, how I waited one day in a state of almost breathless tumescent expectation for their return from a fishing trip, hoping that I might spy on them changing clothes. And in a recurrent dream-fantasy that I somehow know I experienced as a very small child, I remember seeing a line of naked boys pass before as if they were angels come to rescue me, and wanting to possess their bodies in a way I didn't understand.

As a small child, then, same-sex desire was an almost phototropic response, while the knowledge of my damaged physical self was something I strove to obliterate. To oversimplify, I might say that being "gay" was my nature, something I embraced instinctively; being "crippled" was the natural condition I fled from at all cost.

Learning to walk with my first pair of legs, going to school for the first time in second grade, seemed to confirm Dr. Kessler's assertion that I was "totally rehabilitated," but part of the cost of that medical triumph was being set apart. On the first day of school, I sat at my desk holding my breath, clammy with sweat, in a room full of other children, all of whom had known one another since kindergarten. I had never been in a room with so many other children—I'd been socialized among adults. Sister Aloysia announced to the class that here was the new boy and they must all be careful not to knock him over. So of course, on the playground, I didn't play, I talked to the nuns, safe once again among adults. I imagine now that I was an insufferable little prig of a child, "talking to the nuns" instead of playing, but that everyone was too kind to say so because I was, after all . . . disabled.

By then I suspect that talking had already become my first line of defense against the unimaginable, the What-Will-They-Do-To-Me-Next? Damage Control to protect against more trauma. As a very small child I had been acted upon incessantly, prodded, laid bare on tables, flesh exposed, bone cut into. All without preparation or warning. A three- or four-year-old cannot stop adults with words, so I had been unable to talk my way out of the ether mask clapped to my face, my limbs lopped off. But now, a little later—but light years later, too—could I not use speech to alternately fend off and invite, as circumstances warranted?

If I could charm adults, might they leave me alone, abandon their schemes to cut off more of me? But this defense was a delicate balancing act, for I must not call too much attention to myself. I think that's how I became the child who was articulate but who never made demands (who when taken to New York City's biggest toy store, for example, and invited to choose anything, chose the *smallest* thing).

To ask, to demand, to have a will, meant visibility. And visibility was treacherous, the flip side of impotent rage.

If talking offered some chance of holding adults at bay, it promised, conversely, that other children might be invited to forget how different I looked. Talking, if I became adept at it, might deflect their relentless curiosity. If I could entertain them with stories, distract them with the transformative magic of language, might they not stop asking, "What happened to you?"

One day I decided that the "soft carpal mass" of my "rudimentary right hand" resembled the puppet character Kukla on the television show *Kukla, Fran, and Ollie.* I enhanced the resemblance by drawing a face on my hand and adding puppet shows to my repertoire of verbal distraction and seduction. I think this must have been an almost instinctive way of saying, "Before you mock my odd-formed body I will do it myself."

I don't mean to suggest that the small-child me in any way planned a strategy of verbal distraction and seduction. I believe that it evolved as part of a subtle cause-and-effect mechanism that went hand in hand with the development of the creative neuroses that serve the adult me as carapace and defense. None of these responses proves that I had an unhappy childhood. In fact, I am convinced I was, in many ways, a happy child, but crafting happiness took work. Writing the script for happiness implied the existence of places in my own life where I was refused entry. The script dictated that there were things about myself I could not, would not, see.

Then came the mirror. The mirror is puberty, when you see yourself for the first time and imagine, obsessively, how others see you. Like the hunchbacked dwarf who entertains the infanta in Oscar Wilde's fairy tale, "The Birthday of the Infanta," I saw my *self* in a mirror "for the first time." But hormones had pumped into overdrive by then, morphing the dreamy state of generalized eroticism that I'd recognized since infancy into—SEX. So when I looked into the mirror I saw an asymmetrical, limping figure with missing parts. I was appalled. This is how it felt for Adam and Eve to recognize their nakedness, I concluded. This is not a trivial matter of embarrassment. This is the deep stuff: Shame.

But why shame? What ingredient needs to be added to a clear view of the naked self to result in shame? Proof that the world's opinion and the mirror's evidence are congruent. Let me cite three mileposts that measure the territory of shame between the time I began high school and the start of college: (1) I get a summer job in the town library. I overhear the head librarian deciding not to put me at the front desk, for "How would it look?" (2) When I pick up my girlfriend (I knew I was queer but I had no idea what to *do* about it) from her baby-sitting job one summer afternoon, Miriam reports a question from her employer: "Why does your mother let you go out with a boy who looks *like that?*" (3) I fall in love for the first time, with my college roommate—yes, that old cliché. John responds to my agonized confession with a question. "Do you think you'll ever find a man who'll sleep with you?"

Helen V. D. Winter, you old harridan of a librarian, you deserved all of the jokes we made about your name behind your back, but at the age of sixteen I thought you were right. How *would* it look? That's how thoroughly I had absorbed the world's view of me. Miriam, you and I laughed off Mrs. Richbitch's question, but at home that night, I wondered what your mother *did* think. And what *you* thought. Only decades later, discovering by chance that you had turned out to be a lover of women, and therefore might have folded my peculiarities into your own outsider's worldview, did it also occur to me that your Holocaust-survivor parents might have judged my missing limbs from a perspective broader than any spoiled suburban matron's. And John. Dear handsome, blond, pipe-smoking, poetry-spouting, pretentious John, my *beau ideal* of a collegiate lover, yours was the question that mattered most. Yours was the negative assumption, the challenge, which mysteriously engendered hope, for how else would I have had the self-possession to answer you by saying, "Yes. If I can find the right man." Where that glimmer of belief in my *self* came from I have no idea. I do know that I have spent every day of my life since then proving you wrong.

Frustrated by how much I haven't been able to relate (nuances, subtleties, simple facts) and how much more remains to be told, I'll have to speed up the film. I'm twenty now, still smarting from my roommate's question, when at last I am divested of my troublesome virginity. It happens like this. A group of us campus misfits and would-be intellectuals wander through the woods on a peerless fall day. Wally entertains us with tales of his conquests. I am awed not so much by the numbers as by the fact that someone could boast about all the *men* he's slept with. I'm also envious—enraged—that Wally is feasting while I'm starving. As the group breaks up, I push my face into his and snarl, "If you ever develop a taste for the grotesque, let me know!" Two weeks later he calls my bluff. We live together for fifteen years.

I would like to tell you that this ended with Happily Ever After, but like the man who has been starving for too long, I found myself unable to digest all of this rich food. Earlier I had tried to escape the distress of trauma by fleeing from what I saw in the mirror, by disassociating from my body. Now, married to Wally, I add to that tactic. I respond to my sense of shame and powerlessness by cooperating in a relationship where I continue to feel powerless, put-down—abjectly grateful that finally I *have* "found a man who'll sleep with me."

There's one more aspect to the mirroring phenomenon that you need to know about before we continue. I turn away from mirrors in frames, it's true, and for years I also turned away from living mirrors, the disabled people who reflect my reality just as effectively as silvered glass does. I fled from the company of anyone with a limp or a hump or a chair on wheels, anyone with a drag or a drool or a spastic face and, most of all, anyone with missing parts. It's an article of faith with me: I refused to be around disabled people. Because I want to pass. And they reminded me that I can't. Because *they* are who *I* am. They won't let me have my escapist fantasies, dammit, so I'll disappear them.

Occasionally my resolve would exhibit cracks, for example the time, years ago, living in a small town in New Jersey, when I began to notice that my supermarket of choice was frequented by a young man with what I then thought of as an unusually severe case of cerebral palsy. Movement was difficult for him, his features (and his speech, as overheard in the checkout line), seemed to me grievously distorted. At first I put as many aisles between us as I could manage, because I knew that if the normals saw us together, they would realize at once that I was not one of them but was, instead, more like this young man's twin. Even though his eyes held my reflection more clearly than the polished plate glass I carefully avoided looking into, I eventually did start saying "Hi," and "How are you?" when our shopping paths crossed, or when I saw him make his way (struggling, it seemed to me) across a busy intersection. One day a friend told me, "Hey, you know that guy who lives on Elm Street, the one who has so much trouble walking? You'll never guess where I saw him last night. In

Tony's!" Tony's was our small town's single (and part-time) gay bar. So, our twinship was complete, it seemed. That newfound knowledge began to nudge me almost imperceptibly toward the possibility of something more than a fleeting "Hi!" But, in the end, I couldn't take the step. I could not look so steadily into the mirror.

So that's what I did for most of my life. I was the crip equivalent of the House Nigger, the Tom, who seeks to elevate his own status by denying the people who define his deepest reality.

I wish I could tell you precisely, in minute detail, how all of my internal cogs and gears and ratchets began to shift me from dead center, how far too late in my life I've started to stop trying to pass. A new marriage helped immeasurably, a marriage of equals, and maybe something so basic as a change of scene, a move from one coast to the other. Maybe I was simply exhausted from the game, tired of going out of my way to bypass mirror after mirror. Anyhow, I accepted an invitation to write something for a tiny gay disability magazine—the transformative magic of language again, always an effective anodyne for me. But as I accepted another assignment and then another, I found there was no way to continue without engaging the subject directly. How could I write about "them" if I was intent on disappearing them?

I interviewed a couple of disabled gay men and helped one or two of them write articles. I was even able to write a piece about my own ambivalence. Then one day I woke up to find that I had a few crip friends, and although my oldest friend had herself become disabled in midlife, these crips seemed like my very first disabled friends, perhaps because they were men and they were gay—and I had discovered them for myself. I was finding that I could sit at the Café Flore in San Francisco and have coffee with a guy in a wheelchair and (how was this happening?) he didn't give me the creeps anymore. I could even find him . . . sexy, though I still had to fight that old queasy feeling sometimes. Often, in fact. The feeling that being seen with other crips would make me conspicuous, one of *them*. "Yeah," I wanted to acknowledge to the cute, abled passerby when he shot us a questioning glance as he passed the café, "these crips give *me* the creeps, too." Instead, what I can more often imagine saying these days is, "Yeah, well, I still don't always like it, but I *am* one of them. So why don't you just hurry off to the gym before your abs atrophy."

I felt bereft when the tiny magazine folded. There I was, just stepping over a threshold into a big, scary, beautiful, mysterious room when somebody slams the door in my face. With a lot of help and encouragement, I decided I had to build a room of my own. That room turned out to be a Web 'zine called *Bent: A Journal of Cripgay Voices,* where many of the stories you have read in this anthology first appeared. What I try to do at *Bent,* on the simplest level, is give disabled gay men a place to write about their lives. Time and again I've been rewarded with writing that is eloquent, supercharged, blunt, elegant, down-to-earth, poetic—cripgay lives told every which way.

We who are accustomed to being medicalized, analyzed, evaluated, counted off by statistical standards, are tired of being passengers. We are determined to drive this vehicle that is our lives. We do so in *Bent* by the simplest means: telling our stories. As editor, I sometimes suggest a topic, and I often offer help with shaping a piece, but, for the most part, contributors do the choosing as well as the writing. We write about growing up as crips; coming to terms with traumatic injury; surviving depression and attempts at suicide; about what society thinks of us, says about us, says *to* us; we write a lot about body image and we write a lot about sex and love—longing for it, getting it, not getting it.

These recurrent themes all add up to the One Big Theme, our efforts to claim our full humanity. Our stories, as recounted in *Bent,* teach us that society is no help in this endeavor. Society, in fact, will do all it can to beat us bloody. This hard fact is one we should have learned already from the struggles of blacks, women, queers, and crips. Why should cripgay liberation be any different?

The stories in *Bent* are the life stories and poems and essays I needed to read during all those years when I was devoting most of my energy to evading mirrors. Here they are and there seems to be no end to them and their truth telling. I continue with *Bent* because I believe we have no choice but to be one another's allies, because I believe that we can help one another find a way to vent the rage and ameliorate the depression that results from being despised and rejected, and by so doing discover the part of ourselves that refuses to be put down, classified as second-best, disposable, unlovable. As we tell our stories, we are creating a community, "a body of persons having a common history or common social and political interests; a body of persons of common interests scattered through a larger society."

Maybe it's because I never enjoyed such a community that I'm still afraid of it. Yet I want to be a part of it.

Every cripgay story I help tell in *Bent* is part of my own still-uncertain effort to claim my own humanity. Scattered through a larger society, we seek our common interests with little help and few allies. The community we need is one we must build for ourselves, however ambivalent some of us may continue to be about its ultimate shape and the ways and means we use to create it.

SPECIAL 25%-OFF DISCOUNT!

Order a copy of this book with this form or online at:
http://www.haworthpress.com/store/product.asp?sku=4902

QUEER CRIPS

Disabled Gay Men and Their Stories

_____in hardbound at $29.96 (regularly $39.95) (ISBN: 1-56023-456-3)

_____in softbound at $14.96 (regularly $19.95) (ISBN: 1-56023-457-1)

Or order online and use special offer code HEC25 in the shopping cart.

COST OF BOOKS_____

OUTSIDE US/CANADA/
MEXICO: ADD 20%_____

POSTAGE & HANDLING_____
(US: $5.00 for first book & $2.00
for each additional book)
Outside US: $6.00 for first book)
& $2.00 for each additional book)

SUBTOTAL_____

IN CANADA: ADD 7% GST_____

STATE TAX_____
(NY, OH & MN residents, please
add appropriate local sales tax)

FINAL TOTAL_____
(If paying in Canadian funds,
convert using the current
exchange rate, UNESCO
coupons welcome)

☐ **BILL ME LATER:** ($5 service charge will be added)
(Bill-me option is good on US/Canada/Mexico orders only;
not good to jobbers, wholesalers, or subscription agencies.)

☐ Check here if billing address is different from
shipping address and attach purchase order and
billing address information.

Signature_____

☐ **PAYMENT ENCLOSED: $_____**

☐ **PLEASE CHARGE TO MY CREDIT CARD.**

☐ Visa ☐ MasterCard ☐ AmEx ☐ Discover
☐ Diner's Club ☐ Eurocard ☐ JCB

Account # _____

Exp. Date_____

Signature_____

Prices in US dollars and subject to change without notice.

NAME_____

INSTITUTION_____

ADDRESS_____

CITY_____

STATE/ZIP_____

COUNTRY_____ COUNTY (NY residents only)_____

TEL_____ FAX_____

E-MAIL_____

May we use your e-mail address for confirmations and other types of information? ☐ Yes ☐ No
We appreciate receiving your e-mail address and fax number. Haworth would like to e-mail or fax special
discount offers to you, as a preferred customer. **We will never share, rent, or exchange your e-mail address
or fax number.** We regard such actions as an invasion of your privacy.

Order From Your Local Bookstore or Directly From
The Haworth Press, Inc.

10 Alice Street, Binghamton, New York 13904-1580 • USA
TELEPHONE: 1-800-HAWORTH (1-800-429-6784) / Outside US/Canada: (607) 722-5857
FAX: 1-800-895-0582 / Outside US/Canada: (607) 771-0012
E-mailto: orders@haworthpress.com
PLEASE PHOTOCOPY THIS FORM FOR YOUR PERSONAL USE.
http://www.HaworthPress.com   BOF03